Eat This... It'll

Mamma's Italian Home Cooking

and Other Favorites

of Family and Friends

by Dom DeLuise

POCKET BOOKS

New York   London   Toronto   Sydney   Tokyo   Singapore

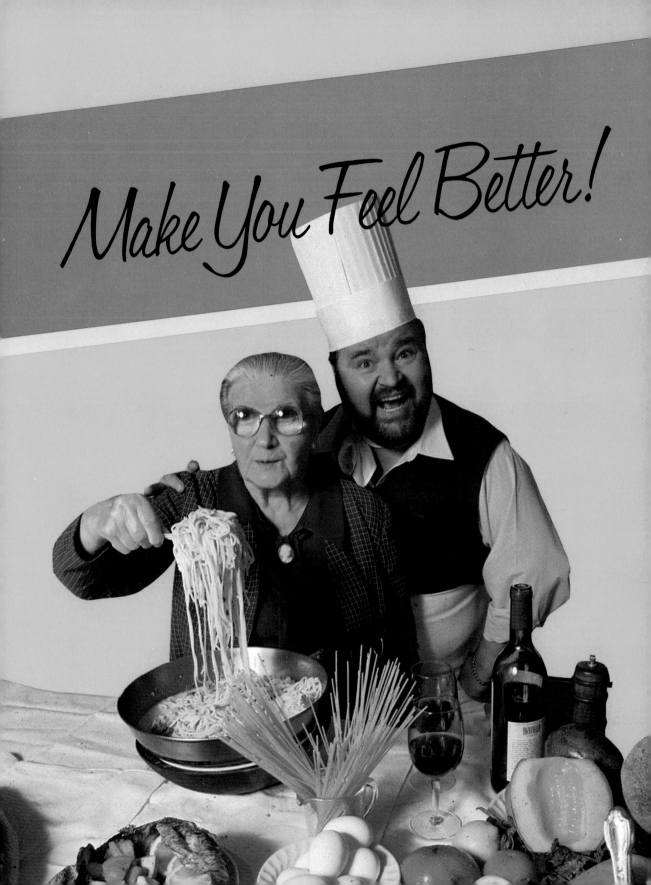

Make You Feel Better!

We have made every effort to trace the ownership of all copyrighted material and to secure permission from copyright holders. In the event of any question arising as to the use of any material, we will be pleased to make the necessary corrections in future printings. Thanks are due to those credited throughout the book, as well to those found on page 139, for permission to use the material indicated.

Acknowledgments

My thanks to Bette Adams, my assistant, who helped me above and beyond the call of duty and who gave her blood, sweat, and tears all through the labor pains and birth of this book.

Carl Furuta was named the best commercial photographer in America in 1983 by *ADWEEK*. When you are working with the best, you know it! Many thanks to Carl and his terrific staff.

Thanks to John Murphy for his great skill and patience.

Illustration on page 198 by Anne Scatto/Levavi and Levavi

POCKET BOOKS, a division of Simon & Schuster Inc.
1230 Avenue of the Americas, New York, N.Y. 10020

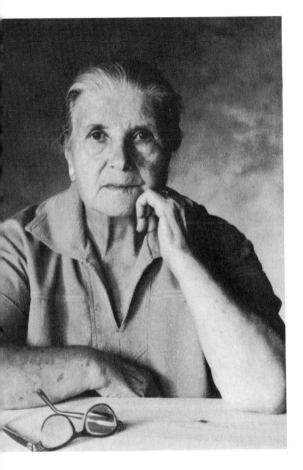

I'd like to dedicate this book to my mother, Vincenza DeStefano DeLuise, who, if you wake up at three o'clock in the morning, would cook for you.

She is the bravest, kindest, smartest person I know, who happens to be a great, subtle Italian cook.

Viva Mamma!

CONTENTS

Preface: Eat This . . . It'll Make You Feel Better   8

Dear Reader   10

Introduction: Look, This Is How I Do It!   12

Me and Salt   19

Me and Grated Cheese   20

Me and Oil   21

Me and Garlic   22

The Feast of St. Ant'eny   23

Soup   27

Salad   46

Egg and Cheese Dishes   60

Vegetables   70

Pasta, Sauces, Rice, and Other Grains   96

     Pasta   99

     Sauces   117

     Rice and Other Grains   136

Poultry and Rabbit   144

Meat   159

Seafood   178

Bread   194

Desserts   208

Index   234

Acknowledgments   239

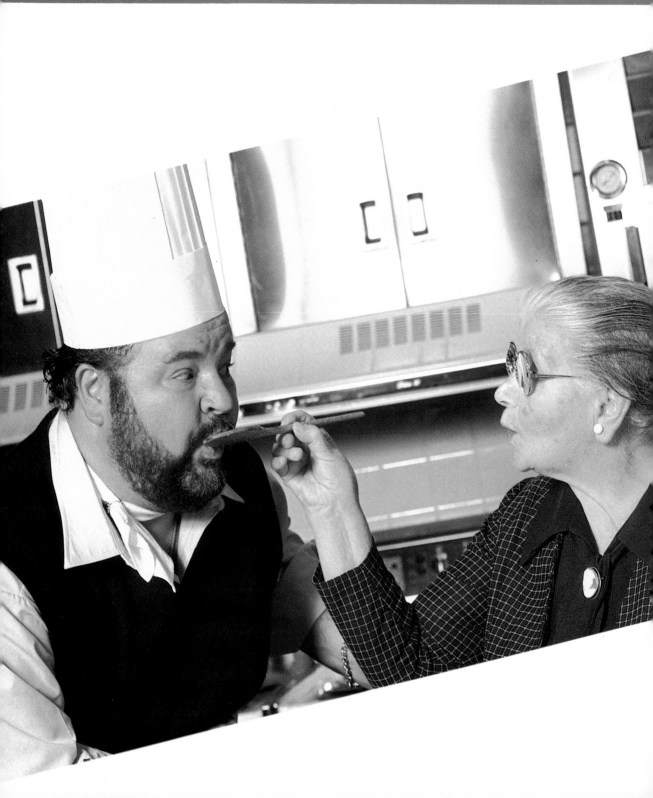

When I was a kid, if I had a fever, had a cold, had a fight, had a fall, had a cut, was depressed, had a disappointment, fell off a truck, woke up with a headache . . . no matter what the situation, my mother's solution was always, "Eat this, it'll make you feel better."

When my father, who had an Italian temper, would yell and scream at me for some childhood indiscretion, my mother was always there with a reassuring cookie, saying, "Eat this, it'll make you feel better."

We used to have *gigantic* meals, at the end of which I would say, "That was great, Ma, it was delicious, but I can't eat another thing . . . I'm going to burst!" That's exactly when my mother would appear with a tray of goodies and say, "Here, eat this, it'll make you feel better."

My philosophy of life had begun! If you have a pain anywhere, inside or out, "Here, eat this, it'll make you feel better."

One of the reasons I wrote this book is because I enjoy making people happy. As a comedian, when I hear the sound of laughter, I am fulfilled. If you enjoy these recipes, and if this book contributes to your happiness in any way, then I'll be thrilled as an author as well. I really hope that you and my book can be friends.

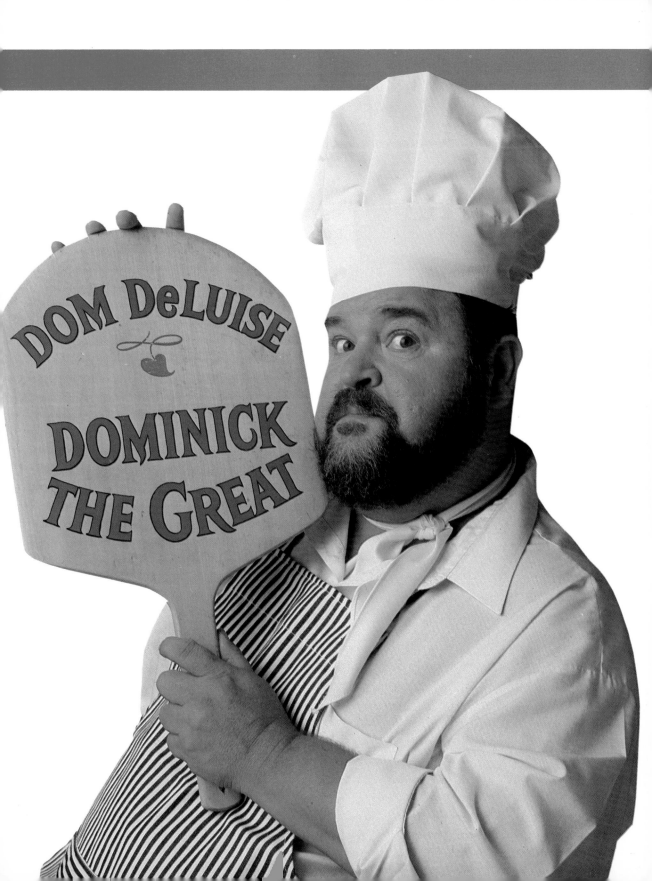

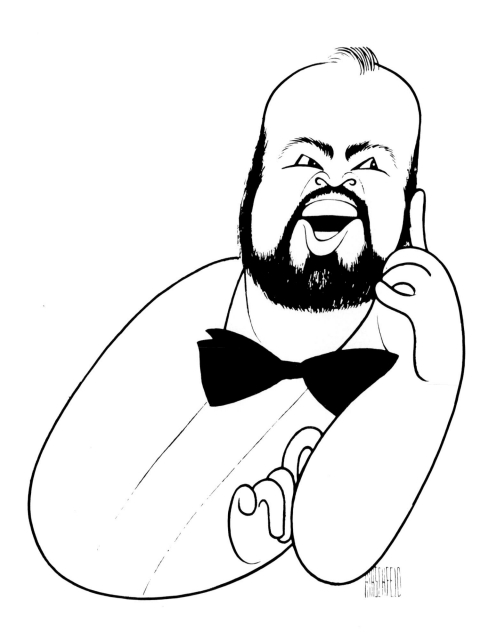

I have a lot of trouble reading books. I tried to read *Gone With the Wind*, but never finished it. I read a lot more of *The Godfather* because Puzo kept talking about the Italian meals the mafioso were having between killings. Seriously, though, while my wife, Carol, is always deep into the latest "self-improvement" book, I have been known to snuggle up with a good cookbook. I *love* to cook for people! If you happen to drop over to my house unexpectedly, it's never too much trouble for me to make a homemade pasta, cooked al dente, topped with a quick homemade sauce.

My mouth "grew up" tasting foods of the neighborhood I lived in, Bensonhurst, Brooklyn, New York. When I was a child my mother made the most delicious Italian peasant dishes, and the more experienced my palate became, the more I realized how special and really terrific her way of cooking was. So I have taken the time to get Mamma's recipes down on paper, along with some of the stories and a lot of the Italian-American traditions that our family enjoyed on Christmas, New Year's, Easter and birthdays.

But the book doesn't stop there. I have eaten in England, France, Belgium, Germany, Holland, my cousin Tessie's house, and when I've tasted something that was absolutely scrumptious, I would grab my host in the kitchen, pin him or her against the wall and force them to tell me exactly what was in the recipe. So . . . if the dish isn't loaded with animal fat, if it doesn't have a lot of salt, but if it *is* loaded with fresh and delicious ingredients so that when people eat it their eyes widen and they say, "Someone kiss me, quick!"—then the recipe is in this book.

Nevertheless, most of the recipes here are Italian, and you can thank my mother for them. Mamma always used phrases like "a pinch of this, some of that," when we collaborated on this book. But her dishes always tasted the same every time she made them. After carefully watching her, I discovered how precise Mamma really was, and took note of her measurements. I also noticed that Mamma cooks with a light touch. She almost never uses the high flame. Her garlic, for instance, is never darker than a golden brown. She simmers gently and she stirs lovingly. Following Mamma's example, you'll find I use only a little oil, mostly for flavor, little or no salt, and lots of garlic. I also follow Mamma's example in being frugal when I cook. For example, I almost never call for a fraction of a vegetable. You'll *never* have a half an onion or a wedge of pepper sitting around the refrigerator. "Waste not, want not" is my mother's credo—and it's mine, too! When I use a can of something, it means juice and all—otherwise I say "drained."

These recipes are fun, fast, healthy, economical and absolutely delicious. But let's face it, folks, most of them are peasant dishes that have been handed down from peasant to peasant, yet also happen to be very much in vogue today. A lot of chic people I know would kill for escarole and beans, which costs only 32 cents a serving. The same was true if you were an Italian growing up in Brooklyn—you might be late picking up your girl because your mom made pasta e fagioli for dinner. Can you imagine? Macaroni and beans coming between you and your future wife?

This collection of recipes represents the best from the best cooks I know: my friends, my family, and most particularly my dear mother—the very best of them all! So I invite you to snuggle up with my cookbook. Happy reading, healthy eating and bon appetite!

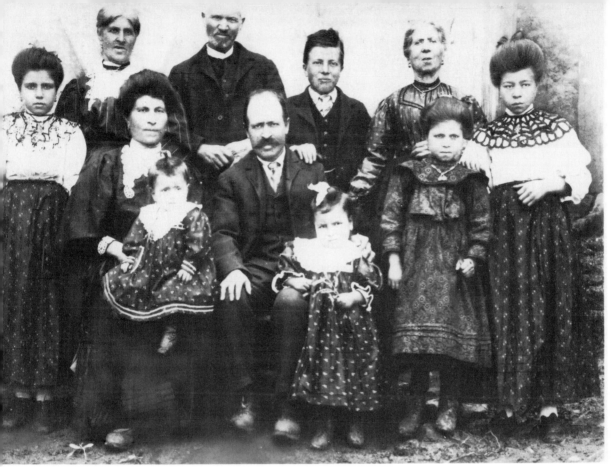

My mother (*left*), age fourteen, standing next to her parents and my great-grandparents.

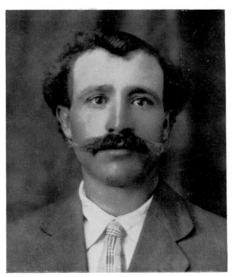
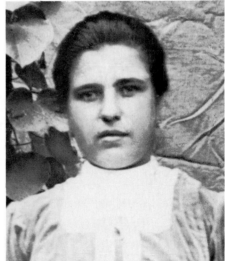

My father and mother when they got married, February 15, 1920. They arrived in New York on September 12, 1920.

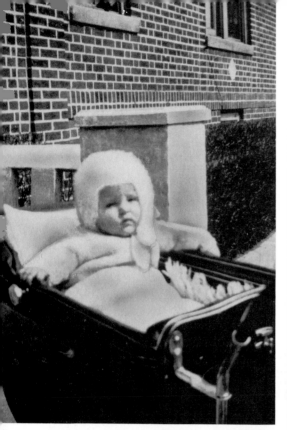

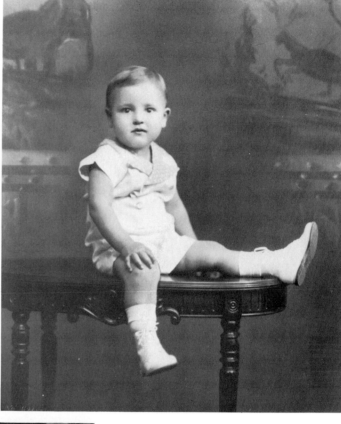

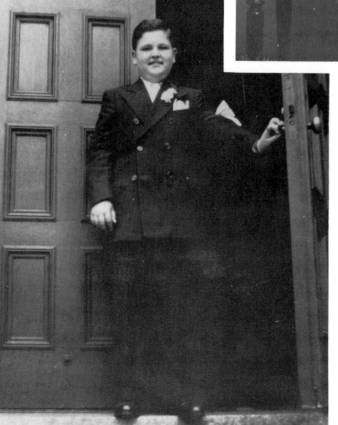

Me!
. . . through the years!

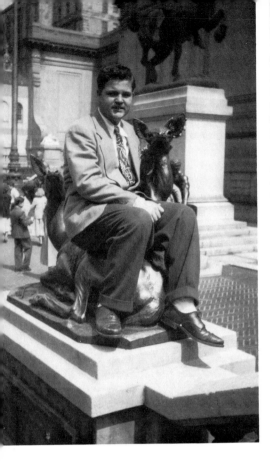

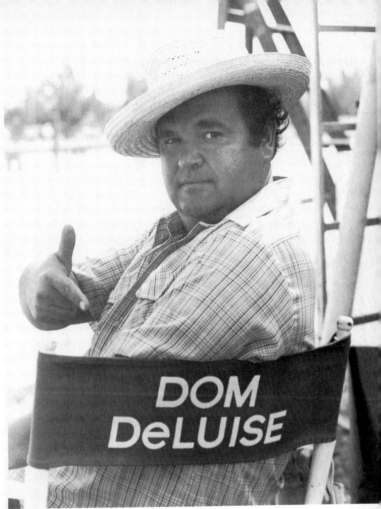

DOM DeLUISE

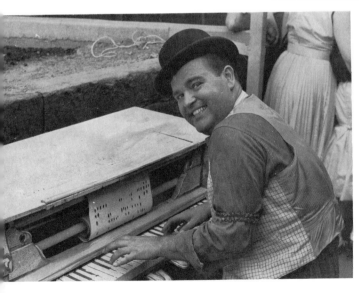

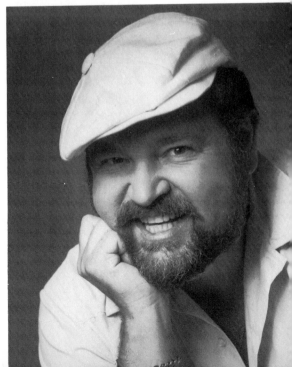

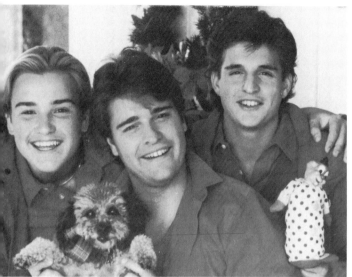

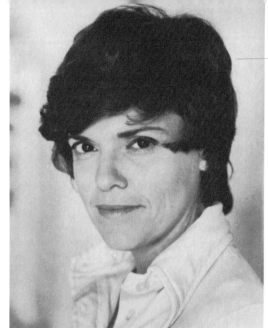

Top left: My three sons, David, Peter, and Michael (*left to right*), and Midnight, Christmas 1986. *Top right:* My sweet Carol. *Bottom left:* Some of my family when we got together for an Easter snack!—1987. *Bottom right:* Me and Mamma.

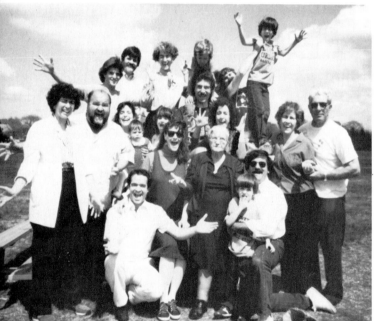

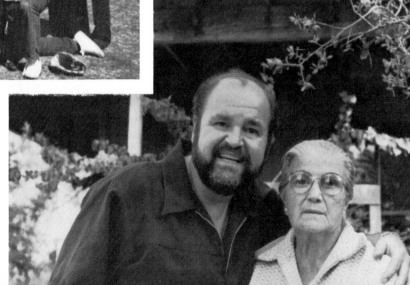

Salt may be good for melting ice in your driveway, but let's face it, it is not very good for *you*—so you won't find much of it in this book. Grated cheese, canned tomatoes, canned broth all have sufficient salt for most of these recipes. Besides, I knew you wouldn't want to muck up the natural tastes of the fresh ingredients we'll be using in the recipes that follow.

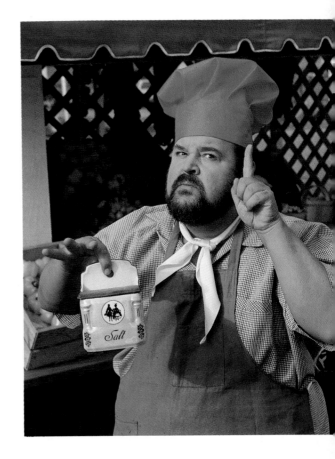

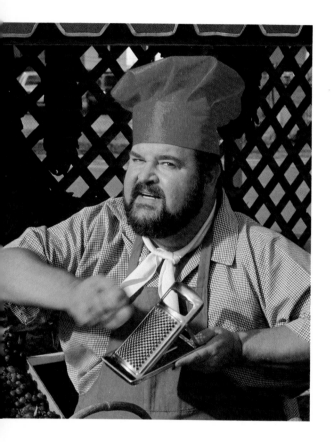

Since it is an important part of many of the dishes here, I urge you to use the best imported cheese for grating. Parmigiano Reggiano is the most popular. But decide for yourself. Do what I do—I go to the Italian store, taste the cheeses, then I buy a piece and have it *freshly grated*. I prefer a combination of Romano and Parmesan, which I keep in an airtight jar in the refrigerator. When a recipe calls for grated cheese, that's what I mean. Of course, you can use any freshly grated Italian cheese you like—I want us to be friends! P.S. You may want to keep a hunk in your refrigerator to grate as needed.

Ah, the flavor of a good olive oil. Fabulous! Truly the work of the gods. And there is new and good news about it as well. The latest findings show that olive oil is monounsaturated—that means it's even better for you than polyunsaturated because it helps break up cholesterol. So flavor is not the only reason we use it; it's also good for us. Besides, I'm so Italian, instead of blood, I feel I have virgin olive oil running in my veins . . . just for flavor!

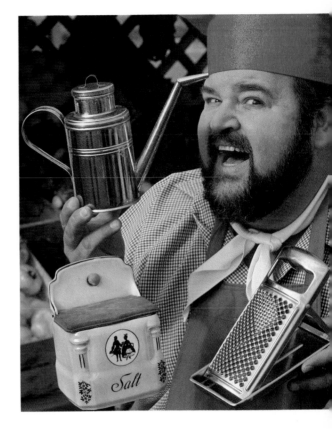

ME AND GARLIC

Somebody once gave me a pillow with the inscription "You Can't Be Too Rich and You Can't Be Too Thin." Oh, yeah? Well, you can't have too much sex—and you can't have too much garlic. But if you have too much garlic—you probably won't have any sex. So, if you are in search of something to embroider on a pillow, don't look at me.

But I feel I should warn you that a lot of the recipes in this book do contain garlic, sometimes a hint, sometimes a lot. I wanted us to have this understanding before any further intimacies.

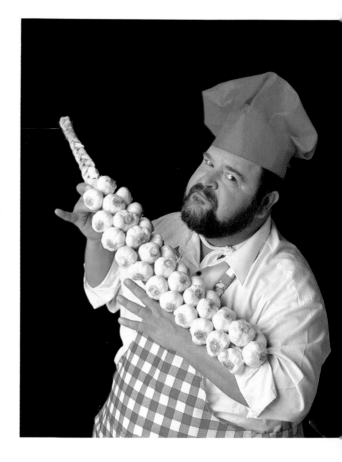

My mother and father were both immigrants from Italy who heard that the streets of America were paved with gold. Sure enough they both came here, and my father got a job *cleaning* those streets of gold (he had a job with the Department of Sanitation for twenty-five years). I grew up in an Italian section . . . Italian! Oh, *please*, some of the names I heard when I was growing up—Salvatore Orena, Dominick Bimbo, Cosmo Infantalino. . . . And these were just the Jews in our neighborhood!

Anyway, our family lived right across the street from a huge Italian church called Regina Pacis, which means Queen of Peace. Once a year all the Italians would get together and celebrate "La Festa di Santo Antonio." Gee, that sounds like a disease, doesn't it? "Look, I got a festa di Santo Antonio." It just means the Feast of St. Anthony. OK. OK. So the whole block would be roped off while the celebrating was done in the street. There was always live music. I remember I used to love to watch my cousin Tessie dancing with her little son Rudy. He would put his small feet on top of her shoes and they would dance in the middle of the street with big smiles on their faces. What joy! Then, just as it was getting dark, they would have a procession through the streets to the church where they would get a BIG Madonna—a life-size statue called a *marone* (a derivation of the word "Madonna") which would be carried by three big guys and one poor little guy who would, of course, get all the weight.

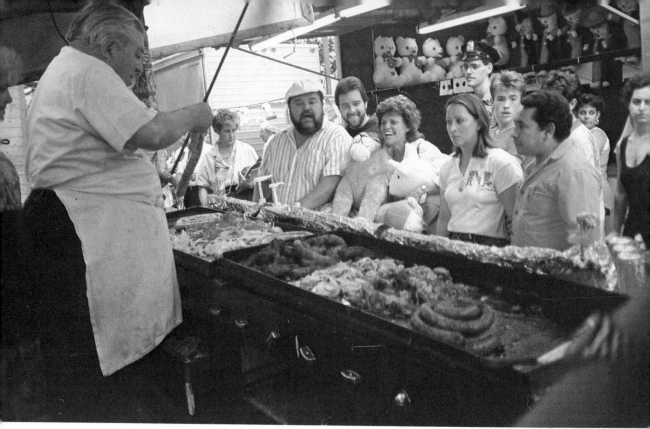

That's me with Father Pat Boyle and Carol, you guessed it, buying sausages at the Feast of St. Ant'eny, 1987.

These four carried the statue up, over and through the crowd, so it looked like it was moving on its own, miraculously gliding through the streets. And as the musicians played their slow, moving music, chills went up my young Italian spine. Our neighborhood band was made up of everyone, it seemed, over eighty, playing mostly trumpets and drums with all their might. Taatatata rah . . . *boom!* It was very moving . . . but I always imagined that poor little guy, staggering under the weight of this tremendous statue moaning, "*Please*, play a little faster. This *marone* is killing me!"

There were games and laughter and food. Food! Wonderful, fragrant, delicious food: clams on the half shell that would be pulled out of barrels of chopped ice; pizza; calzone; oh, and my favorite, a sausage sandwich. This burly guy would take steaming sausages with peppers and onions and shove them into hot Italian bread. When you bite into one of these sandwiches you have to lean forward because the juice runs down your neck.

It was after the beer, and the three quarters of an hour it took me to finish that incredible sandwich, that I always made my way over to the zeppoli man. He would make a flour, water and yeast mixture, then take a little between his fingers and drop it into bubbling hot fat. These zeppoli make a wonderful noise as they turn a golden brown . . . sssssssssssssssssssss! While they were still piping hot, his wife, a tiny lady named Mariache, would drop them into a paper bag followed by ten shakes of powdered sugar. Finally I'd hand her a quarter and she'd hand me this steaming bag of goodies. I couldn't wait to reach in with two fingers and pull out a hot crispy treat covered with snowy white powdered sugar. Anyone who's ever eaten zeppoli at an Italian street festival knows that a little powdered sugar always gets on the end of your nose. It's part of the fun!

As the afternoon came to a close—and this was the most fun of all! —when I was ready to go home, I'd face in the direction of my house, tighten my ass and . . . *brrrrr*, I'd slide home! Then, when I came to a corner and had to turn, I'd just raise my left arm and . . . *brrrrr*, turn right! Or my right arm to *brrrrr* turn left. I imagine I looked just like the marone moving, gliding miraculously through the Brooklyn streets. . . . Amazing, really, it wasn't just food, it was also transportation.

But enough of tender memories. On to soup! *Avanti!*

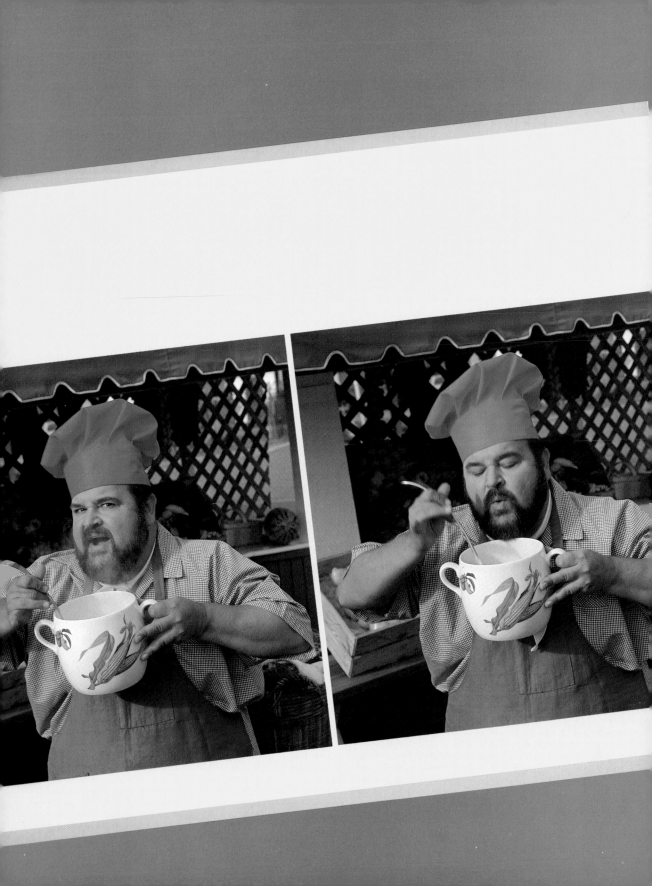

Soup

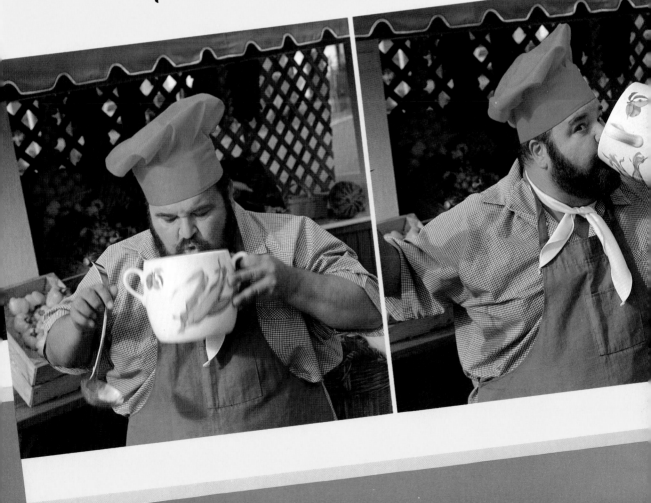

BRRR, COLD

When I was eight years old, growing up in Brooklyn, I used to dread waking up in winter to a cold house, when the tile on the kitchen floor would be really cold. But on those mornings when it was 30 degrees outside, I'd run lickety-split to the kitchen and there Mamma had the hot oven door open and she'd be warming up my underwear and shirt. I knew that would be the day I could expect one of my favorite hot soups on Mamma's stove when I got home. Warm underwear when I was a kid and hot, bracing soups on frosted days— just part of what makes me thankful for my sweet mother.

MAMMA'S ESCAROLE SOUP

When I was in Italy visiting my mother's hometown of Spinosa, I had lunch at my Aunt Madeline's farm. This wonderful, tiny woman (she's five foot nothing) insisted that the simple soup she was going to serve was a peasant dish. She kept apologizing for it! Of course it was extraordinary, just like the escarole soup my mother makes, but this was extra delicious served with the hot bread that came out of her stone oven.

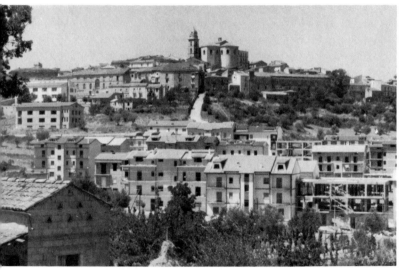

My folks' hometown, Spinosa, Italy. They were married in Saint Mary's Church at the top of the town.

2 tablespoons olive oil
2 garlic cloves, minced
1 onion, chopped
2 carrots, sliced
1 potato, peeled, diced (optional)
2 cups chicken broth
2 heads of escarole, well washed and coarsely cut

In a large saucepan, heat olive oil and gently brown garlic. Add onion, carrots and, if using, the potato (this breaks up and helps thicken the soup), and then after 1 minute, the broth. Add escarole, cover and let come to a boil. Lower to simmer for 1 hour. For soupier soup, use a little broth or water.

Variation: You can add spareribs, and/or a couple of Italian sausages at the same time as the garlic and brown the meat well. Then add everything else.

Serve in soup bowls and sprinkle with grated cheese. Have lots of hot Italian bread on the table.

SERVES 6–8.

ESCAROLE AND BEANS

Italians make a tiny funny happy noise way down in their throats every time you say the words "Escarole and beans." If a food can be friendly, this is one of the "friendliest." *Emiss!*

1 cup chicken broth
1 large head escarole (well washed and coarsely cut)
2 tablespoons olive oil
2 garlic cloves, minced
1 15-oz. can cannellini beans
4 fresh basil leaves, cut up

In a large saucepan place chicken broth and escarole, bring to a boil and simmer for an hour. Gently brown the garlic in the oil, then add cannellini beans with their liquid and heat thoroughly. Combine with escarole and let simmer for 10–20 minutes. Stir carefully with wooden spoon. This should have a soupy consistency (add a little more broth, or water, if necessary).

This is excellent with hot pepper flakes, grated cheese, and hot Italian bread.

SERVES 4.

MAMMA'S LENTIL SOUP

As a young kid, I thought lentils were one of the strangest and most useless things in the whole world. *Yuk!* In fact, when I was putting this book together, every grownup that I asked hated lentils when they were kids. So the moral of this story is: Never serve this soup to anyone under thirty!

1 pound lentils
4 cups chicken broth
3 cups water
2 tablespoons olive oil

2 garlic cloves, minced
4 carrots, diced
1 16-oz. can of crushed tomatoes
  (optional)

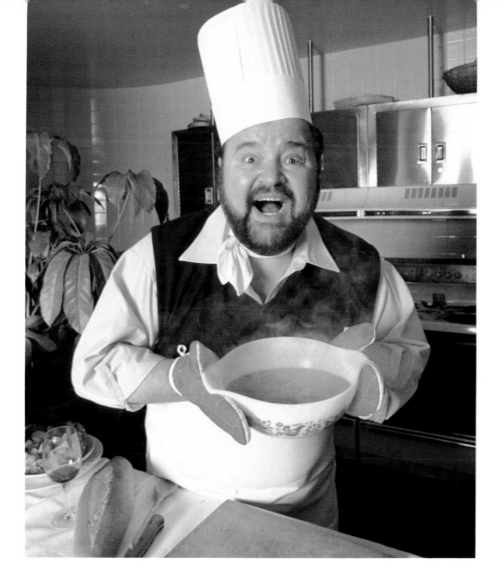

In a large soup pot put lentils, broth, and water. Bring to a boil and simmer for 1 hour and 15 minutes.

In a small pan, gently fry the garlic in the oil until golden brown. Add this to the cooking lentils, along with the carrots. If you like a tomato taste, add the tomatoes. Simmer for 30 minutes more, or until lentils are very tender.

Option: Add ½ pound of cooked ditalini, or cooked spaghetti broken into 2-inch pieces

or: 1 cup cooked white or brown rice.

Serve with grated cheese and hot Italian bread.

SERVES 8–10.

MAMMA'S STRACCIATELLE WITH TINY MEATBALLS

I always loved this soup because it has so many different textures and colors. Stracciatelle means "torn rags," which is what the eggs look like when you stir them into the hot broth. Just know that this soup takes a little more time because of the meatballs, but it's really worth the little extra effort, and it's great to snuggle up to on cold winter nights.

Soup:
1   quart chicken broth
2   cups water
½   cup pastina
1   teaspoon fresh parsley, chopped
1   carrot, sliced thin
½   pound spinach (just leafy part, julienne cut)

Meatball Mixture:
½   pound lean beef
1   egg
2   teaspoons flavored bread crumbs
1   teaspoon grated cheese
2   teaspoons fresh parsley, chopped
1   small onion, minced

2   eggs
*   grated cheese*

In a soup pot, combine soup ingredients and bring to a low boil. Mix meat ingredients in a bowl, make tiny meatballs, and drop into boiling broth mixture.

In a small bowl, beat 2 eggs. With a wooden spoon, stir soup as you slowly drop in the eggs, stirring constantly. Remove from heat. Cover and let stand for 2 minutes.

Serve with grated cheese.

SERVES 6–8.

P.R. SOUP
(Potato Rice Soup)

When I was seven years old, I went to P. S. 187 elementary school in Brooklyn. Every lunch hour I would walk home, and when my mother made this soup for me, I couldn't walk back! Seriously, though, during the Depression this soup was very popular, since it cost about 11 cents to make, and it costs not much more than that today. Still, it's healthy family fare. My kids love it!

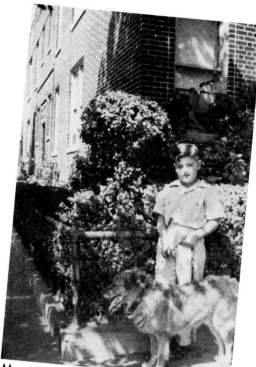

Me, age nine, and Princey in front of our house.

1 *garlic clove*
4 *tablespoons olive oil*
1 *medium onion, chopped*
1 *medium potato, peeled and diced*
1 *cup Italian rice (or your favorite rice will do)*
2 *cups chicken broth*
2 *cups water*
1 *tablespoon fresh parsley, chopped*
1 *tablespoon grated Parmesan cheese*

Gently sauté garlic clove in oil until golden brown. Add onion, potato, rice, broth, water, and parsley. Stir, bring to boil and let simmer for 1 hour, stirring occasionally.

Just before serving, stir in the grated cheese.

Important: This is best served immediately with additional cheese sprinkled on top of each serving.

SERVES 4.

VERONICA'S LAKE

Our friend Veronica Chambers is particularly imaginative in the kitchen. This soup, for instance, evolved from a recipe for sauce— sauce for broiled fish, that is. When I first tasted it Veronica challenged me to guess the ingredients, so I chose every fruit and vegetable except (you guessed it!) the ones below. P.S. I told you this comes from a sauce—but I've renamed it in honor of the obvious!

2   *quarts of chicken stock*
3   *green apples, peeled, cored and chopped*
2   *onions, chopped*
8–10 *carrots, chopped*
½   *cup cream or milk*

In the chicken stock, cook the apples, onions, and carrots for about 1 hour, or until very tender. In a food processor or a blender, process until smooth. Add cream or milk and serve hot. Or serve it cold and call it "Ice Capades!" This also works great as a sauce over broiled fish.

SERVES 8. MAYBE MORE! IT'S WONDERFUL TO HAVE LEFTOVERS, SO USE YOUR IMAGINATION.

MAMMA'S FRIDAY NIGHT HEARTY FISH SOUP

When I was a kid, Fridays were still meatless days for Catholics, but no one in our house complained when Mamma served this. Warning: I have to tell you, there may be happy moaning and groaning after you've dished this up.

Note: Other kinds of fish can be substituted, according to what is available fresh from the market.

2   *tablespoons olive oil*
1   *onion, chopped*
4   *cloves garlic, minced*

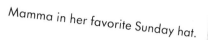

Mamma in her favorite Sunday hat.

2   celery stalks, chopped
2   carrots, sliced
1   green pepper, chopped
2   28-oz. cans tomatoes, crushed
1   16-oz. can tomato sauce
1   6-oz. bottle clam juice
3   medium potatoes, peeled and diced
½   teaspoon pepper
1   teaspoon oregano
4   fresh basil leaves, torn up
½   pound halibut, cut into bite-sized pieces
½   pound sole, cut into bite-sized pieces
½   pound red snapper, cut into bite-sized pieces
1   cup dry white wine
3–4 tablespoons chopped fresh parsley
5–6 fresh basil leaves, chopped, for garnish

Place oil in a large pot, and sauté onion, garlic, celery, carrots and green pepper, just until al dente.

Add tomatoes, tomato sauce, clam juice, and potatoes. Cook over medium heat for 5 minutes. Add pepper, oregano, and basil. Cover and simmer for 20 minutes, or until potatoes are done.

Add fish and wine, cover and continue simmering for 10 minutes. Sprinkle with chopped parsley and/or additional fresh basil before serving.

Delicious with hot crusty bread!

SERVES 6–8.

MEL BROOKS' RED CLAM CHOWDER

Mel Brooks also grew up in Brooklyn and has an affinity for Italian clothes, Italian food and Italian women—like my good friend Anna Maria Italiano (in "real life" she's known as Anne Bancroft). Anne is married to Mel Brooks, who's become very "Italianized" over the years. The four of us have shared a lot of meatballs together. Mel loves pasta e fagioli, zucchini frittata, and marinara sauce on capelli d'angeli, but he once cooked a red clam chowder that made *this* Italian sit up and take notice. I must admit that when Mel made it for us we had fresh clams that we got from the bay on Fire Island. Don't let that stop you, however, because we did add canned clams. (We just didn't tell anybody.)

Me and Mel Brooks by the sea—by the beautiful sea!

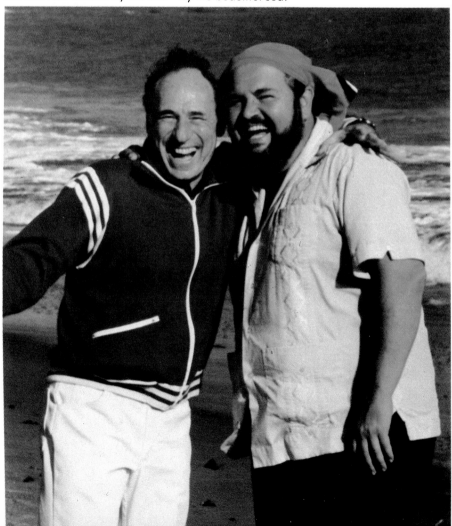

4　strips bacon, cut into 1-inch pieces
2　tablespoons olive oil
4　garlic cloves, minced
1　large onion, chopped
1　medium green pepper, chopped
4　medium potatoes, peeled and diced
4　carrots, diced
2　celery stalks, diced
1　10-oz. can kernel corn
1　28-oz. can crushed tomatoes
2　tablespoons tomato paste
2　6-oz. bottles clam juice
1　cup white wine
4　cups water
½　teaspoon oregano
¼　teaspoon thyme
¼　teaspoon freshly ground pepper
2　teaspoons chopped fresh parsley
2　bay leaves
6　10-oz. cans minced clams (or 4 pounds fresh clams)

In a large pot, gently brown bacon. Add olive oil and sauté garlic and onion until golden brown. Add all other ingredients except clams. Stir, bring to a boil, then reduce to a simmer for 1 hour and 15 minutes. Fifteen minutes before serving add clams.

Serve with hot bread and beer. It's great at any time and if it's cold outside, it's better!

SERVES 10–12.

GAZPACHO

When we first arrived in California, Carol and I rented a beach house in Malibu with our infant son, Peter. We felt like novices in new surroundings. After observing us for two weeks, the lady next door informed us that we were "beach people," a real compliment from Malibuans. Edna McHugh has been our friend for twenty years, and we've always marveled at what a skilled and gracious hostess she is. Carol and I have spent some incredible evenings at her home, with some of the most interesting people in Hollywood. She is a great cook and a chocoholic (author of *Chocolate Kicks*), and also happens to be one of the legendary Eddie Cantor's five daughters.

1	small red onion	$\frac{1}{2}$	teaspoon oregano
1	small green pepper	1	pint V-8 juice
2	cucumbers	1	pint tomato juice
2	hard-cooked eggs	3	tablespoons lime juice
1	garlic clove, crushed	$1\frac{1}{2}$	tablespoons wine vinegar
2	tablespoons salad oil	$1\frac{1}{2}$	teaspoons Worcestershire sauce
$\frac{1}{8}$	teaspoon black pepper	2	drops Tabasco sauce
$\frac{1}{2}$	teaspoon dry mustard		

Mince onion very fine in a wooden bowl. Add green pepper and chop fine. Add peeled and coarsely chopped cucumbers.

Chop hard-cooked eggs in a small bowl and add garlic, oil, pepper, mustard and oregano. Mix well and add to chopped vegetables.

Combine V-8 juice, tomato juice, lime juice, vinegar, Worcestershire sauce and Tabasco in a large pitcher.

Add the rest of the ingredients to pitcher. Mix well and chill thoroughly.

SERVES 4–6.

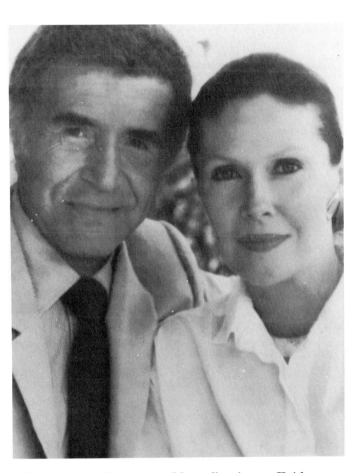

Dom with the Montalbans

Carol and I were at Ricardo and Georgiana Montalban's one Friday night with Burt Reynolds and Loni Anderson. Standing in the center of their living room, we could see the Hollywood lights through the windows twinkling in the night. The view was breathtaking. While we were having drinks Georgiana served these raw vegetables cut into the tiniest, most "civilized" slivers you've ever seen in your life! Now when *I* cut a vegetable, I want it to fit in your mouth. She cuts them, they fit between your *teeth!* Georgiana knows me very well so she completely understands and laughs when she sees me taking six celery sticks at a time.

As you can imagine, Georgiana is a superb cook, and that night she served the most incredible-tasting soup, which I just had to share with you here:

GEORGIANA'S TORTILLA SOUP

1   *large chicken, 4 or 5 pounds*
1   *onion, chopped*
1   *carrot, chopped*
3   *stalks of celery, chopped*
    fresh parsley
12 *corn tortillas*
¼   *cup cilantro, chopped*
1   *avocado, peeled, sliced, and sprinkled with lemon juice*
½   *pound grated Monterey Jack cheese*

Cook the chicken in water to cover for 1½ hours or until tender. Remove the chicken and put the stock in the refrigerator overnight. The next day, remove the fat from the surface. Remove chicken from bones, cut into pieces and put the meat aside. Discard bones.

To the chicken stock, add onions, carrot, celery, and parsley and bring to a boil. Lower heat and simmer until vegetables are done, then add deboned chicken to heat through. Meanwhile, wrap 12 tortillas in foil and gently heat in a 350-degree oven for 15 minutes. Stack 3 tortillas at a time and cut them into ½-inch strips. Ladle the hot soup with chicken pieces into soup bowls, add tortilla strips to each bowl, and top with freshly chopped cilantro and a slice or two of avocado.

Sprinkle top of each serving with grated cheese. It looks almost as good as it tastes!

SERVES 8.

JULANN'S FAT-FREE, HEARTY MUSHROOM BARLEY SOUP

I was the very first guest on the Merv Griffin television show back in 1961. It was at that time that I met Merv's wife, Julann Griffin. We have been good friends ever since. Julann is a very unique woman. She makes her own soap, she has kept bees, she has even been known to make beer in a bathtub! She was the president of the First Women's Bank of California, she plays a mean game of tennis, and she even invented the game "Jeopardy" that Merv produces for television. Julann is a very funny lady, and I have laughed till I cried with her. I've also just cried. She is a fabulous friend, a great cook, and is very concerned with eating healthfully. I have had some of Julann's wonderful, fat-free, hearty soups, and I know you'll love this one as much as I do. (If you'd like this soup a little less "hearty," add more chicken broth and/or tomato juice to your taste.)

1½	cups barley
3	tomatoes, chopped
2	carrots, chopped
1	medium onion, chopped
2	garlic cloves, minced
6	cups chicken stock
2	cups tomato juice
4	fresh sweet basil leaves, chopped
½	teaspoon oregano
10–15	mushrooms, thinly sliced
	pepper to taste
	lowfat yogurt

In a soup pot combine barley, tomatoes, carrots, onion, garlic, chicken stock, tomato juice and herbs. Stir. Bring to a boil. Lower heat, and cover, but not completely—leave lid slightly askew. Stir occasionally. Let soup simmer 1 hour, then stir in the mushrooms. Add pepper and let simmer 1 more hour. Ladle into hot soup bowls and top each with a spoonful of yogurt.

SERVES 8–10.

Dinner at the White House

When my sister Anne invites me to dinner, I say, "Great!" When my mother invites me to dinner I say, "All right!" because I know it's going to be delicious. Those invitations are no problem. But when you get a letter from Washington, D.C., asking you to have dinner at the White House as the guest of the President and Mrs. Reagan, it's pretty hard to keep your cool. The invitation was still warm when I called my mother 3,000 miles away in Brooklyn to tell her. She couldn't believe her "baby" was going to eat at the White House. She was tickled pink!

When the evening came, Carol and I clutched each other's hands as we approached the magnificent entrance hall of the White House, which was, by that time, crowded with guests. Almost immediately, the Marine band began playing "Hail to the Chief," and, to tumultuous applause, in walked the President and Mrs. Reagan, all smiles and looking wonderful. Standing in the receiving line, I pinched myself hard just to make sure this was all really *real!* As the line progressed, we became more and more nervous, but when it was our turn to meet them, the President and Mrs. Reagan could not have made us feel more welcome. Mrs. Reagan was so gracious . . . but so tiny! I figured my lunch weighed more than she did! You can imagine the two of us standing side by side. Quite a sight! It was a great moment.

When everyone picked up their table assignments I felt bad because Carol was at table seven and I was at table number one . . . surely the President's table. But it was when dinner was announced and all the guests moved into the East Room that I saw Carol seated at the table with the President. I was seated at a table with Pat Boone! (That was OK. I love milk and cookies. Sigh.) On my left was a newspaperwoman, and on my right was a regal-looking diplomat who said, "Good evening, my name is Count Kerestesi and I am the Ambassador from Vienna, Austria." So I said, "Hello, my name is Dom DeLuise and I am a comedian from Brooklyn, New York." I had a feeling it was all going to be downhill from there.

Mrs. Reagan had just purchased new White House china and there had been a lot of publicity about it, but when I lifted my dish in order to examine every detail, the newspaperwoman sitting next to me said, "Oh, you're sooo tacky." I couldn't resist: it was time for a little fun.

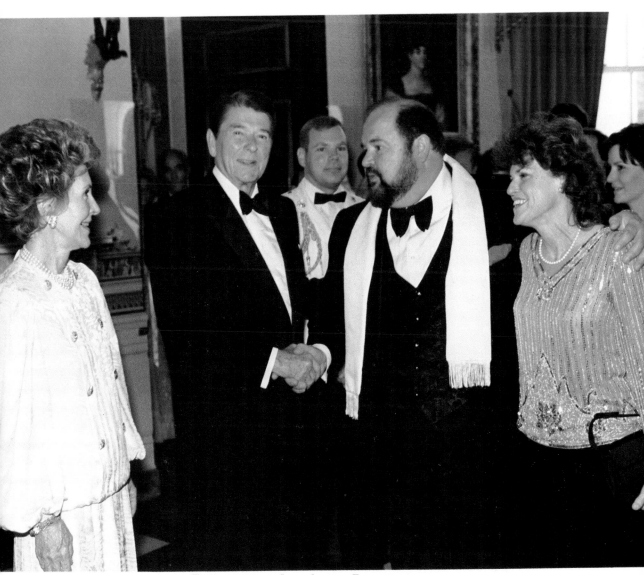

Dear Dom – It was great to be with you.
and Carol Warmest Regard & Friendship,
Ronald Reagan

In front of each guest was a beautifully engraved dinner menu listing soup, squab, braised fennel, carrots and pastries. I lowered my glasses to the end of my nose, looked at the waiter and inquired in my best British accent, "What's fresh today?" "You are!" said the reporter. Then everybody really laughed!

After dinner, a Marine informed Carol and me that Mrs. Reagan would appreciate it if we came over and talked to her and the President. *If* we had the time. If we had time—hah! We ran over and had a wonderful chat for about 20 minutes—wow!!!

Shortly after dessert, the President and Mrs. Reagan said good night and we guests had a chance to dance and walk about the White House. I took some matches that said "The President's House"; I took some napkins that said "The White House"; I took some jelly beans (okay, okay, so I took a lot of jelly beans); and the last thing was a gift from the bartender: a small bottle of champagne with a White House label. Carol and I were among the last to leave as a circle of security men encouraged the guests down the staircase. The souvenirs made so much noise in my pockets—clink! clunk! squash! clink!—as I went down the stairs that I was surprised they didn't call me back for a full body search!

I had heard that Mrs. Reagan was a marvelous cook, so when we were speaking to her that evening I took the opportunity to ask if she wouldn't mind giving me some recipes for this cookbook, and damn if she didn't say yes. I don't know about the President, but as far as I'm concerned, Nancy Reagan is cookin' with gas!

NANCY REAGAN'S ONION WINE SOUP

4   tablespoons butter
5   large onions, chopped
5   cups beef broth
1   celery stalk, chopped
1   large potato, peeled and chopped
1   cup dry white wine
1   tablespoon vinegar
2   teaspoons sugar
1   cup light cream
1   teaspoon minced parsley
   pepper

Melt butter in large saucepan. Add chopped onions and gently sauté (about 10 minutes). Add beef broth, celery and potato. Bring to a boil. Cover and simmer for 30 minutes.

Puree mixture in a blender. Return to saucepan and add wine, vinegar and sugar. Bring to a boil and simmer 5 minutes. Stir in cream, parsley and pepper to taste. Heat thoroughly, being sure not to boil so the cream won't curdle.

SERVES 6–8.

Salad

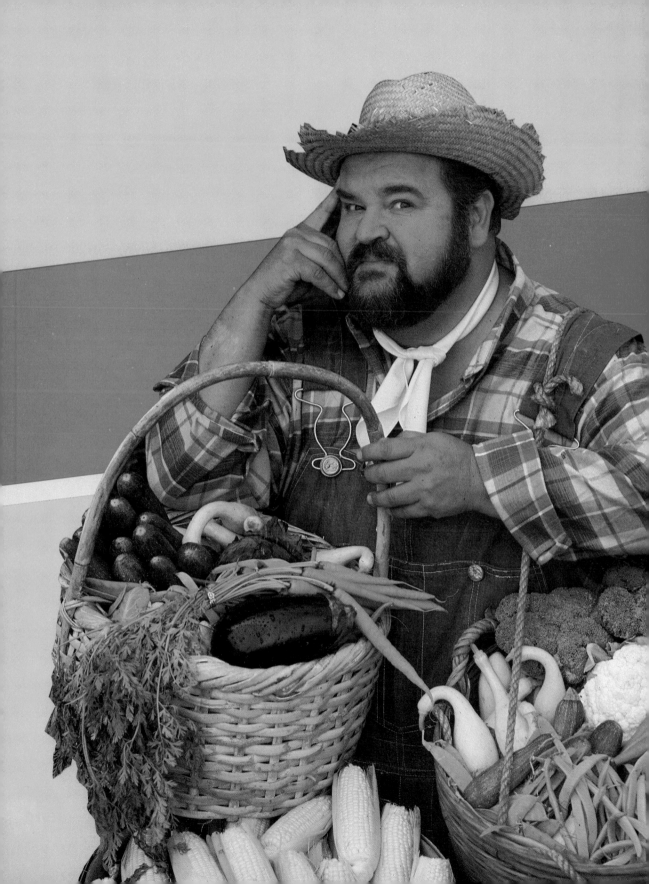

I'm crazy about Italian opera and opera singers in general, particularly tenors. Luciano Pavarotti and Plácido Domingo are both so exciting to my Italian ears, I can't tell you. So you can imagine how thrilled I was when Carol presented me with tickets to a Pavarotti concert at Lincoln Center for my forty-eighth birthday. That night came and we were running a little late so I knew we wouldn't have time for supper—but when I saw the hot-dog man on the street, I figured we'd surely have time for *him*. Picture this: Carol and I dressed to the nines, standing on a New York street corner gobbling up our hot dogs with mustard, sauerkraut, a little bit of hot pepper and an ice-cold Yoo-Hoo. We enjoyed our "dinner," and made it to the theater just in time to hear Luciano's velvet tones. He was magnificent! Thousands of people stood and cheered. His singing brought tears to my eyes and a lump in my throat. I figured I must really have loved his singing . . . either that or I put too much mustard and sauerkraut on my hot dog!

After the performance, Carol and I went to a salad bar and tried to eat light. I love salad and it's very good for you—especially if you have tears in your eyes or lumps in your throat from the world's greatest Italian tenor . . . or too many hot dogs!

Brothers at heart—me and Pavarotti. What a thrill!

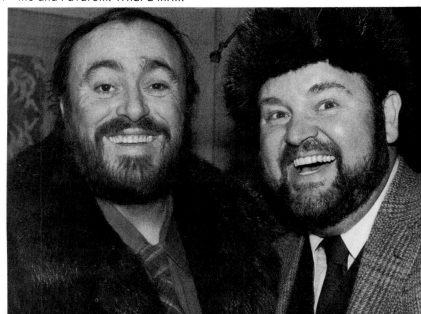

TOMATO AND MOZZARELLA SALAD

My best most favorite breakfast is sliced tomato with fresh basil on toasted Italian bread. For this, I will follow you anywhere!

6   *large tomatoes, sliced*
8   *ounces mozzarella cheese*
1   *purple onion, sliced (optional)*
12 *whole fresh basil leaves*

Dressing:

3   *tablespoons olive oil*
3   *tablespoons red wine vinegar*
1   *garlic clove, minced*
3   *fresh basil leaves, coarsely chopped*
¼   *teaspoon oregano*
    pepper

On a bed of lettuce, arrange tomatoes, cheese, onion, if using, and basil. Mix all dressing ingredients together and pour on top. Garnish with sprigs of parsley, if desired.

My roasted peppers on page 79 are a wonderful addition to this salad.

SERVES 8.

Note: I sometimes simply serve a tomato slice topped with a slice of mozzarella, topped with fresh basil leaves and sprinkled with a little olive oil. Great at buffets and I never have leftovers.

VIVA MONTALBAN SALAD

If it's possible for a salad to be a class act, this one certainly is—
because it's created by Georgiana Montalban, the classiest lady I
know! Ah, Georgiana, Ricardo has all the luck!

 1 *head Bibb lettuce*
 1 *head radicchio*
 6 *artichoke hearts, cooked (see Artichoke Hearts, page 51)*
 6 *tablespoons sour cream*
 6 *tablespoons caviar*
    grated onion or chopped hard-cooked egg
    lemon, cut into wedges
12 *radishes*
12 *asparagus spears, raw (if very young) or parboiled*
12 *black olives*
12 *carrot sticks*
 1 *cucumber, peeled and sliced*
    vinaigrette sauce

On each round, flat salad dish, make a bed of Bibb lettuce, with the
curly edges of the lettuce going all around the outside of the dish. In
the middle of the dish, place 2 radicchio leaves and an artichoke heart,
with a dollop of sour cream, on which you place a tablespoon of your
favorite black caviar. (The colors so far are great.) Sprinkle the caviar
with little grated onion or chopped hard-boiled egg, whichever turns
you on. Lean a lemon wedge against the bottoms of the artichoke
hearts.

Around this beautiful and tasty center, place the other vegetables
2 by 2: 2 radishes, 2 asparagus spears, 2 olives, etc. Sprinkle the
vegetables with some vinaigrette dressing just before serving.

SERVES 6.

ARTICHOKE HEARTS

Artichoke hearts are delicious, healthful, look very impressive on the table and are extremely versatile. Once my agent Merritt Blake's wife even made lasagne with thin slices of artichoke hearts instead of pasta and it was one of the lightest meals I'd ever eaten. So here's the basic recipe—fabulous served hot or cold.

2   *tablespoons flour*
    water
5   *cups chicken broth*
2   *lemons*
8   *large artichokes*

To make a cooking liquid that will keep the artichokes from turning brown, place the flour in a large saucepan, gradually beat in 1 cup of cold water, stir in the 5 cups of broth, and the juice of 1 lemon, bring to a boil, stirring, then remove from heat.

Cut stems off artichokes, trim the ends, peel, and drop into a bowl of cold water with the juice of 1 lemon. One by one, break leaves off artichokes, bending leaves back upon themselves all around, until you come to the crown, or the light-colored inner leaves. Cut off the darker green tops of the inner leaves. Carefully trim the bases of the artichokes to remove the dark green part, rubbing bases frequently with cut lemon to prevent darkening. Drop each heart into the bowl of cooking liquid along with the stems. When all the artichokes are prepared, simmer hearts and stems about 30 minutes, or until just tender when pierced with a knife. Don't overcook. Drain the artichokes and refresh under cold water to prevent further cooking and restore color.

You can serve these as a vegetable, or use in salad, or surprise yourself.

SERVES 8.

DOM'S CAESAR SALAD

The original Caesar salad did not include anchovies, but they have somehow become a traditional ingredient. I've reverted back to the original!

1   *head romaine lettuce*
1   *clove garlic, cut in half*
3   *tablespoons fresh lemon juice*
5   *tablespoons olive oil*
1   *teaspoon Dijon-style mustard*
    dash of freshly ground pepper
1   *egg yolk*
¾   *cup seasoned croutons*
2   *tablespoons grated cheese*

Wash lettuce and tear into large pieces. Rub garlic halves around inside of a large wooden salad bowl and discard garlic.

In salad bowl, combine lemon juice, oil, mustard and pepper. Add egg yolk and mix well. Add the lettuce, croutons, and Parmesan, and toss lightly. Sprinkle each serving with additional Parmesan cheese.

SERVES 4–6.

DOM'S CHINESE CHICKEN SALAD

I serve this in the biggest bowl I can find. Make more than you need and stand back!

1   *2–3-pound chicken, poached in 1 cup water and 1 cup white wine
     (remove the meat, discard bones and skin, and slice the meat in
     finger pieces)—or, if you prefer, use 4 or 5 chicken breasts,
     poached and boned*
1   *large head iceberg lettuce (about 6 cups), thinly shredded*
3   *green onions (including tops), thinly sliced*
2   *celery stalks, thinly sliced*
1   *can water chestnuts, drained and sliced*
2   *cups bean sprouts*
1/2 *cup coarsely chopped cilantro
     Dom's Chinese Chicken Salad Dressing (page 54)*
2–3 *cups Deep-Fried Bean Threads or Rice Sticks (directions below)*
1/4 *cup sesame seeds*
1/2 *cup cashew nuts*

In a salad bowl, mix together chicken, lettuce, onion, celery, water chestnuts, bean sprouts and cilantro.

Drizzle Dom's Chinese Chicken Salad Dressing over chicken mixture and toss lightly. Add bean threads or rice sticks and toss again, even more lightly.

Top with sesame seeds and cashew nuts.

SERVES 6.

Deep-Fried Bean Threads or Rice Sticks

Pour salad oil (about 2 inches) into a wok or deep pan on medium-high heat. Drop in one bean thread or rice stick. If it expands at once, the oil is ready. Cook a small handful at a time. As noodles puff and expand, push them down into the oil with a slotted spoon, then turn over the entire mass to be sure all are cooked. When noodles stop crackling (about 30 seconds), remove with a strainer and drain on paper towels.

DOM'S CHINESE CHICKEN SALAD DRESSING

When I was in the middle of writing this book, I thought I had the best Chinese chicken salad dressing in town. Then one day, Carol and I went to see my good friend Bill McCutcheon at the Ahmanson Theater in "Light Up the Sky." After the show, Bill and his wife, Anne, and Carol and I went to a restaurant, and I realized that I was wrong. We all agreed that they served the best Chinese chicken salad dressing we'd ever tasted. I called the waiter over and promised him a small house in Connecticut if he'd get me the recipe, and here it is, folks!

6   *cups seasoned rice vinegar*
32 *cups water*
3   *pounds sugar*
2   *cups plum sauce*
¾   *cup soy sauce*
1   *ounce fresh ginger, minced fine*
1   *garlic clove, peeled, left whole*
1   *tablespoon sesame oil*

Heat vinegar. Add water and sugar and bring to a boil to dissolve sugar. Remove from heat. Add plum sauce, soy sauce, ginger, garlic and oil. Refrigerate overnight.

Now, if you are expecting over 400 people for lunch, that recipe is perfect, but I've broken it down for smaller groups.

⅔   *cup seasoned rice vinegar*
2½ *cups water*
½   *cup sugar*
¼   *cup plum sauce*
⅛   *cup soy sauce*
1   *tablespoon fresh ginger, minced or grated*
1   *garlic clove, peeled, left whole*
¼   *tablespoon sesame oil*

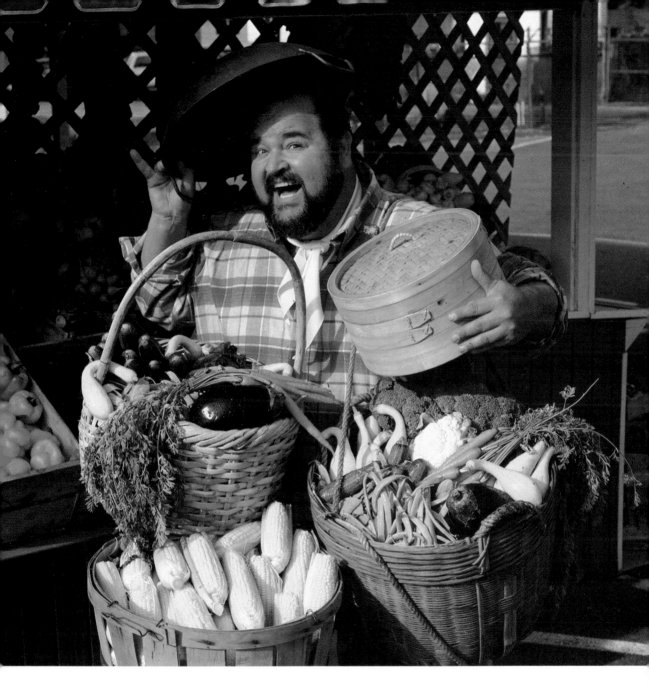

Heat vinegar. Add water and sugar and bring to a boil to dissolve
sugar. Remove from heat. Add plum sauce, soy sauce, ginger, garlic,
and oil. Refrigerate overnight.

MAKES JUST UNDER A QUART.

DOM'S SEAFOOD PASTA SALAD

This is easy, fast and a crowd pleaser. Prepare ahead of time so you will be able to chit and chat and mingle and dingle along with your guests. No problem.

1   *pound shrimp, peeled and deveined*
1   *pound scallops*
2   *pounds cheese tortellini*
½   *cup olive oil*
½   *cup fresh lemon juice*
1   *cup fresh basil leaves*
1   *garlic clove, minced*
½   *cup grated cheese*
     pepper
     fresh basil leaves, for garnish

Boil the shrimp and scallops for 3 to 4 minutes, until *just* cooked. Drain and let cool. Cook tortellini until al dente, drain and let cool. Combine olive oil, lemon juice, basil leaves, minced garlic and grated cheese in a food processor or blender. Toss all ingredients together. Add pepper to taste and garnish with more fresh basil leaves.

SERVES 8–12 OR WORKS *GREAT* AT A BUFFET.

SALVATORE'S SISTER SALLY'S SENSATIONAL SUMMER SALAD

When I was a teenager, my best friend was Salvatore Orena. I loved his family. His mom made the best spaghetti sauce on 11th Avenue. His sister Bubbles, also a marvelous cook, made this incredible salad for us (but I had to change her name to Sally, otherwise it would've screwed up the title). This is a salad that does take some time, but you'll get such a great response when you serve it, you'll know it was all worth it.

1   small bunch broccoli, cut into florets
½   small head cauliflower, cut into florets
6   carrots, sliced
1   green pepper, cut in chunks
1   red pepper, cut in chunks
10 green beans, cut into 1-inch pieces
3   celery stalks, sliced
3   medium zucchini, sliced
½   cup peas
8   large mushrooms, quartered
1   red onion, sliced in rings

Dressing:
1   cup mayonnaise
2   tablespoons safflower oil
6   tablespoons lemon juice
½   teaspoon fresh or dried tarragon
1   teaspoon fresh dill
1   tablespoon fresh parsley,
    chopped

whole lettuce leaves
parsley sprigs for garnish

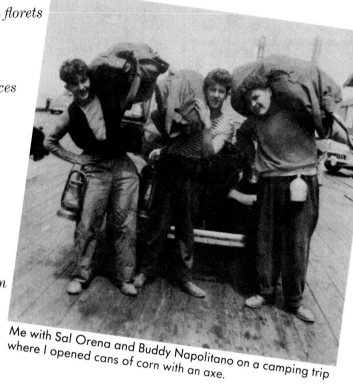

Me with Sal Orena and Buddy Napolitano on a camping trip where I opened cans of corn with an axe.

Add broccoli, cauliflower, carrots, peppers, green beans, celery to a pot in which 2 cups of water are boiling, and cover. Steam lightly for 5 minutes or until barely done. At this point add zucchini, peas and mushrooms and steam a little longer. Drain and cool.

In a separate bowl, mix together the ingredients for the dressing.

Gently toss salad with mayonnaise mixture. Top with overlapping onion rings and garnish with parsley sprigs. Store in refrigerator. Serve on a bed of lettuce leaves.

SERVES 12–14.

It's great on a buffet table. It's sure to satisfy saints and sinners simultaneously—I swear.

EAST-WEST ASPARAGUS SALAD

A very easy dish which always makes those eyebrows go up—and the olive oil and sugar are great together, for sure.

1   *pound fresh asparagus*
2   *tablespoons soy sauce*
1   *teaspoon brown sugar*
1   *tablespoon olive oil*

Cut or break off the tough bottoms of the spears. Cut spears into 2-inch pieces. Drop into a pot of boiling water and simmer 2 minutes, or just until tender. Do not overcook. Drain and rinse immediately under cold running water until the asparagus are cool. Drain well. Place asparagus in a bowl and add the soy sauce, sugar, and oil. Mix well. Serve on a bed of lettuce.

SERVES 4.

MY VINAIGRETTE DRESSING (ITALIAN STYLE)

This is a good all-around dressing. It's great for marinating meat, fish or fowl, and it's great on salads as well.

½ *cup olive oil*
½ *cup wine vinegar*
1 *tablespoon Dijon mustard*
1 *teaspoon fresh dill*
1 *scallion, minced*
¼ *teaspoon oregano*
¼ *teaspoon thyme*
2 *fresh basil leaves, torn up, or* ¼ *teaspoon dried*
    freshly ground pepper
2 *tablespoons lemon juice*

Put all ingredients in a jar, cap and shake well. If you'd like to make Creamy Vinaigrette, add 2 tablespoons of sour cream to all of the above ingredients and then shake well.

MAKES 1¼ CUPS.

Egg and Cheese Dishes

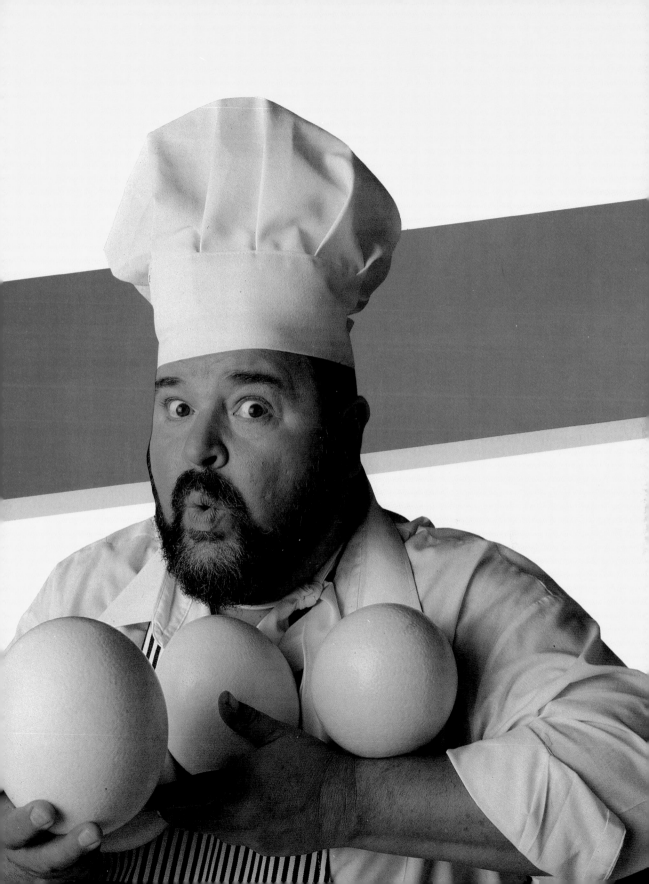

FIT FOR A KING

The first time I ever cooked I was about eight years old. It was on a day I found myself alone in the house. Papa was hunting for deer in New Jersey, my mother was doing a novena at the church, my sister and brother were both in school—but *I* was ready for lunch. The fact that Mamma was not at her post, ready, willing and able to cook anything that was not moving, was what made this day different from other days. I'll show them, I said to myself. *I'll do it alone.* Anyway, I ended up throwing two slices of mortadella and two eggs into a frying pan; then I sprinkled the top with slices of mozzarella. I toasted Italian bread, and on a side dish put slices of beefsteak tomatoes dribbled with a little olive oil. To my delight and astonishment, I realized that the combination of these things tasted like it was fit for a king!

Mamma also does wonderful things with eggs. She combines them with sausages, and with peppers, onions, potatoes, and in fact almost any vegetable. Following in her footsteps, I am now known all along the Western seaboard for the shameless things that I do with eggs. (Some say I am the fastest yolk in the West!)

THE ITALIAN SCRAMBLE
(Soft and Fluffy)

This omelet is delicious for a Sunday brunch or a midnight snack. Since it contains everything but the kitchen sink, it's a wonderful way to clean out your vegetable drawer.

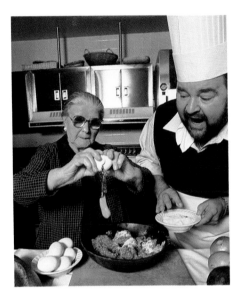

1   *tablespoon olive oil*
1   *medium potato, cubed*
½   *pound sweet Italian sausages*
1   *small onion, chopped*
1   *small green pepper, chopped*
1   *small red pepper, chopped*
8   *eggs*
2   *tablespoons milk*
⅛   *teaspoon oregano*
1   *firm, ripe tomato, seeded and chopped*
¼   *cup shredded mozzarella*
¼   *cup grated cheese*
     chopped fresh parsley for garnish
     hot Italian bread

Heat olive oil in a large frying pan and add the potato; cook over medium heat, stirring occasionally. Remove sausage casings and crumble the meat into the frying pan, cooking and stirring until lightly browned. Add onion and peppers and cook until onion is limp and the potato cubes are done.

Beat the eggs together with the milk and oregano. All at once, add the tomatoes, egg mixture and mozzarella to the frying pan. Lower the heat and cook, stirring lightly until eggs are soft and fluffy, and I do mean soft and fluffy . . . not hard and stiff. The mozarrella should stretch and bring you great happiness. Top with grated cheese and parsley and serve with hot Italian bread.

SERVES 4–6.

DOM'S EGGS ALLA DIAVOLO

This could be a Sunday supper, but for some this devilish recipe can visit anytime!

1 *onion, chopped*
1 *tablespoon olive oil*
1 *28-oz. can crushed tomatoes*
½ *teaspoon pepper*
6 *eggs*
6 *teaspoons grated cheese*
6 *fresh basil leaves torn into large pieces*
   Tabasco sauce (optional)

In a large skillet gently sauté onion in the olive oil until translucent, add tomatoes and pepper—stir—when tomatoes are bubbling, break eggs into the sauce and top each egg with 1 teaspoon of the grated cheese. Cover and simmer 4 or 5 minutes—just until egg whites are firm. Spoon tomato sauce around eggs. Garnish with fresh basil and a few drops of Tabasco sauce, if you like. Serve immediately with hot bread.

SERVES 3.

A FRITTATA FOR JULIA CHILD

A few years ago I was asked to do "Good Morning America" with Julia Child. If you think I was nervous the day I got married, you can imagine what it was like to cook for Julia Child! But she turned out to be a real fun lady and a good sport. She could tell I was a little nervous cooking in front of her, so when we began breaking eggs she began throwing the shells over her shoulder! When I followed suit, I realized that Julia not only broke the eggs, she "broke the ice"!

4   *tablespoons olive oil*
2   *garlic cloves, minced*
1   *onion, cut in thin crescents*
1   *potato, thinly sliced to cook quickly (optional)*
1   *red pepper, sliced*
1   *green pepper, sliced*
6–8 *mushrooms, quartered*
6–8 *eggs*
1   *cup grated mozzarella or Monterey Jack*
     fresh basil leaves

Put 3 tablespoons of oil in a large iron skillet and slowly sauté the garlic, onion, potato, and the peppers until thoroughly tender. Add mushrooms and cook 2 minutes.

In a large mixing bowl, combine eggs and grated cheese. Then pour the vegetable mixture into the mixing bowl and beat together. Reheat the skillet, adding 1 tablespoon of oil. Pour the egg-and-vegetable mixture into the skillet. Shake the pan and cook *slowly* over low heat for 10 to 15 minutes, covered. If center isn't done, place under the broiler for 1 minute—watching carefully that it doesn't burn. Take the pan and shake it to loosen, and slip the frittata onto a large dish.

Garnish with fresh basil leaves. Cut into pie wedges. Serve with a green salad and large slices of beefsteak tomatoes. You have a great, light Italian lunch fit for a "Child."

P.S. It's good cold, it's good room temperature, it's good reheated . . . it's just good!

SERVES 6.

ARTICHOKE FRITTATA

Artichokes have a great flavor. I like them alone as a vegetable, and even cold the next day. And if you are out of artichokes, when making this recipe, try your favorite green vegetable—like asparagus or broccoli—in their place and see what happens.

8–10 *frozen artichoke hearts, drained*
2   *garlic cloves, minced*
1   *medium onion, cut in crescents*
3   *tablespoons olive oil*
6   *eggs*
1/2   *cup milk*
1/4   *teaspoon dried oregano*
1/8   *teaspoon pepper*
1   *cup shredded mozzarella cheese*
1/2   *cup grated cheese*
       fresh basil leaves

Cook artichoke hearts, following directions on package, until tender, cut in half and set aside. In a medium-size iron skillet, sauté the garlic and onion in 2 tablespoons of olive oil until golden brown. In a large mixing bowl, combine the eggs, milk, oregano, pepper, shredded mozzarella and 1/4 cup of the grated cheese. Add the cooked garlic-and-onion mixture. Mix well.

Reheat the skillet as you add 1 tablespoon of olive oil and arrange the cut artichoke hearts face down and placed evenly in the skillet. Add the entire contents of the mixing bowl and lower the heat. Shake the pan, cover and cook slowly for 10 to 15 minutes. Sprinkle the top with the remaining 1/4 cup of grated cheese and place under the broiler, until the frittata is puffed and golden brown. Take the pan and shake it to loosen the frittata, and slip it onto a serving dish.

Garnish with fresh basil leaves. Cut into pie wedges. Serve with slices of beefsteak tomatoes and a salad.

SERVES 6–8.

ANNA BANANA'S ITALIAN SAUSAGE PIE

In my neighborhood a lot of people had nicknames. My brother was Nick the Prince 'cause he was tall and handsome. Then there was Frankie Fish, Liver Lips Louise, and Anna Banana. Anna and I've been friends for twenty-five years and I'm still calling her Anna Banana. Better yet, she's still answering! Ladies and gents . . . it gives me great pleasure to present . . . Anna Banana's Sausage Pie.

Piecrust:

3 eggs
2 tablespoons oil
2 tablespoons water

2 cups flour
1 teaspoon baking powder

Beat eggs, oil and water together and set aside. Sift flour and baking powder in a large bowl. Make a well in the center, and gradually add egg mixture. Blend until the mixture forms a large ball. Set aside, covered, for 10 minutes. Knead until smooth, place back into the bowl, cover and refrigerate until ready to use.

Filling:

3 pounds sweet Italian sausage
3 eggs
3 cups ricotta cheese

1 pound grated mozzarella cheese
½ cup fresh parsley
dash black pepper

4 hard-cooked eggs, shelled and thinly sliced
1 egg

Simmer sausage in a large frying pan with water just covering the bottom of the pan, until sausage is brown and water is gone. When cool, slice on an angle, about ¼ inch thick. Set aside. Combine next 5 ingredients and mix well.

Roll out half the pastry dough to fit the bottom of a springform pan. Put the filling into pastry-lined pan and then place the sliced hard-cooked eggs on the filling. Roll the remaining pastry dough into a circle and cover the top, folding the edges of the crust over the rim; seal and pinch crusts together. Slit a few steam vents in the top. Beat remaining egg with about 1 tablespoon of water and brush the top of the pie. Bake for 35–40 minutes at 350 degrees. Serve warm or cold.

MAKES ONE 10-INCH SPRINGFORM, 3 INCHES DEEP.

Croquettes to Phone Home About

When I grew up we did not have a phone. Finally, when I was fifteen years old, we got our very own telephone, and all the DeLuises were very excited. Anytime the phone rang, the entire family would stampede to the living room, stare at the phone and yell, "Ma, it's the phone!" until Mamma picked it up.

One day I left Brooklyn to go to Manhattan with friends to see a movie. I was going to be late for dinner and it was an "Egg Croquette" night, which was one of my favorite dishes. I wanted my mother to know that I was going to come home late, so I called home and my father miraculously picked up the receiver. You understand, this was the very first time he had spoken on our new telephone. "Hello, who here?" he shouted.

"Hello, Pa, it's Dom," I said.

"Doma no here."

"I know, Pa," I said. *"I'm* Dom."

He said, "Doma's go to New York."

And I said, "Pa, this *is* Dom."

"I tella once, I tella again, Doma ina New York, God damn–a!" he shouted.

"Pa, this is Dom, I'm in New York and . . ."

"Dom ina New York, yes, I justa tella you that!"

I gave up. "Okay, okay, I'll get Dom later."

And my father, now calm, said, "OK, I tella him you call. Goodbye."

When I got home my dad said, "Dom, you frienda call. The phone no work so good, but I speaka loud and clear and tella him you in New York!"

"Who was it, Pop?"

"You friend," he said with a smile, "but no worry, he gonna call again!"

I said, "Thanks, Pop." I sat down to eat; Mamma had saved me Egg Croquettes after all and I was too busy eating them to explain.

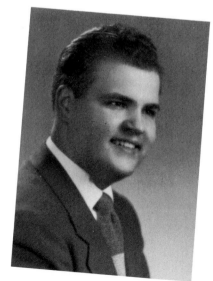

VINCENZA'S EGG CROQUETTES

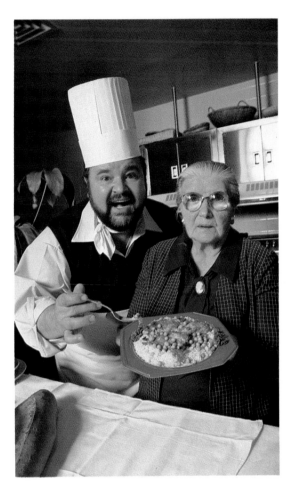

4   *eggs, beaten*
½   *cup bread crumbs*
½   *cup grated cheese*
5   *tablespoons chopped*
    parsley
4   *tablespoons olive oil*
1   *onion, chopped*
1   *garlic clove, minced*
1   *8-oz. can tomato sauce*
½   *cup water*
1   *cup peas (frozen, fresh,*
    or canned)
1   *cup of rice cooked in*
    2 cups of chicken broth

Combine eggs, bread crumbs, cheese and parsley in a bowl. Pour oil into a deep saucepan, and sauté the chopped onion and garlic. Add the tomato sauce, water and peas. Bring to a boil, reduce to a simmer.

While above is getting hot, form dumplings out of the egg mixture by using a soup spoon. Carefully place the croquettes in the sauce one by one. Wet spoon in hot sauce before forming next croquette. *Do not stir! Do not touch!* Croquettes take time to set! Cover and cook over low heat for about 30 minutes. Serve over cooked rice.

SERVES 4.

Vegetables

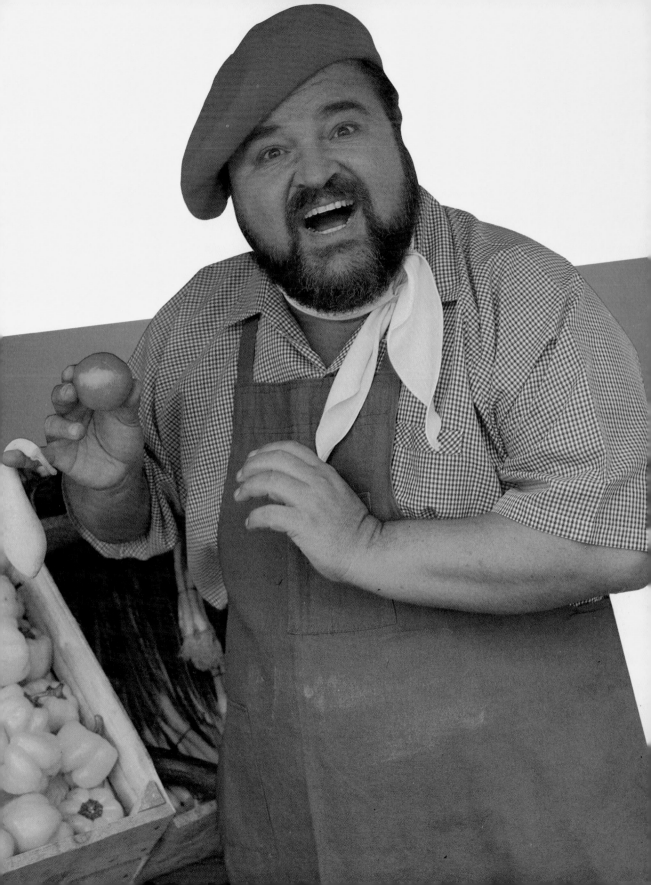

Shouldn't Stew Have Meat in It?

When I was growing up in Brooklyn, a lot of our social life was connected with the church and holidays and weddings and confirmations. Life seemed wonderful and full. We'd eat "fancy" on those occasions, but at home during the week our family would eat very simple dishes—those peasant dishes that have turned out to be chic today: escarole and beans, lentil soup, frittatas, string beans and tomatoes, spinach and potatoes—very little meat. Mamma would often cook vegetable stew, for example, and it was delicious. Then one day when I was over at a friend's house I noticed his mother making her stew with *meat* in it. "How long has this been going on?" I wondered. It was then that I realized my mamma's vegetable stew was unique. It was also very economical; and, at that time, if you did it on Friday, very religious.

You see, vegetables were the staple around my house. Even today, I'd rather be seen with a bunch of broccoli than a side of beef!

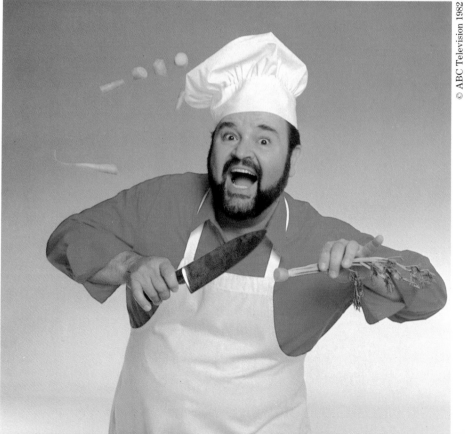

VEGETABLE STEW

4	*tablespoons olive oil*
4	*garlic cloves, minced*
2	*onions, sliced*
4	*carrots, peeled and cut into 1-inch pieces*
2	*celery stalks cut in ½-inch pieces*
2	*large potatoes, peeled and cut into 1½-inch pieces*
2	*cups of fresh peas*
1	*18-oz. can of stewed tomatoes*
1	*28-oz. can of crushed tomatoes*
1	*teaspoon oregano*
8	*leaves of fresh basil coarsely chopped*
10–12	*mushrooms, quartered*
	pepper

In a large pan gently heat the oil, add the garlic and onions, and sauté for a few minutes, then add the carrots, celery, potatoes and peas. Add both kinds of tomatoes, pepper, oregano and basil, and simmer for 40 minutes, until the carrots are just tender. Then add mushrooms and allow the stew to cook for 2 to 3 minutes more. Delicious with hot bread.

SERVES 6.

MAMMA'S SPINACH AND POTATOES IN BROTH

I don't know why it took me a long time to appreciate this terrific dish of my mother's. Spinach never had it so good!

2 tablespoons olive oil
2 garlic cloves, minced
1 cup chicken broth
1 cup water
4 medium potatoes, peeled, quartered, and parboiled
2 pounds spinach, well washed

Place oil in a large saucepan and gently brown garlic. To the pot add chicken broth, water, and the potatoes. Add spinach. Cover and cook 15 minutes. You'll notice spinach has collaped to almost nothing.

This is a soupy mixture but the garlic, potatoes, and spinach mingle together and you won't want to leave a drop of this behind. Just have plenty of hot Italian bread around so you can get it all.

SERVES 4.

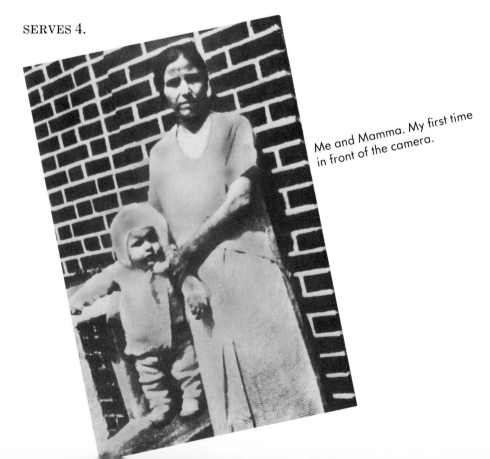

Me and Mamma. My first time in front of the camera.

MY SISTER ANNE'S STRING BEANS

Now you can make any vegetable "Italian" with these ingredients—just like my sister.

1   *pound string beans, cut in 2-inch pieces*
    or *broccoli florets*
    or *asparagus spears*
    or *mix some of each*
1   *tablespoon olive oil*
¼   *cup seasoned bread crumbs*
¼   *cup grated cheese*
    pepper
    fresh basil leaves, coarsely chopped

Steam string beans (or whichever vegetable you choose) for 5 minutes and drain. Heat oil in pan and sauté vegetable(s) for 3 minutes. Add bread crumbs, cheese, and pepper. Toss together thoroughly. Garnish with fresh basil.

SERVES 4–6.

Me and Anne, my favorite sister—also my only sister. I had no choice.

Anna Maria Italiano's Potatoes and Fagioli

Anne Bancroft is a dear friend of mine, a fellow Italian who grew up in the Bronx. She is one of the most talented actresses in the world, and has an Academy Award to prove it. She directed a movie that I starred in called *Fatso*, in which there were a lot of references to our Italian background, humor and eating habits. Anne is married to one of the funniest men in the world, Mel Brooks, who is Jewish. There is very little difference between Jews and Italians. The Jews have matzo balls and the Italians have meatballs. They both love their families, and they both love to laugh, yell and scream a lot. Carol and I and Mel and Anne often spend an evening eating matzo meatballs, talking about our families, laughing, yelling and screaming . . . a *lot!*

I went to Anne Bancroft's house with a tape recorder in order to get this recipe straight. Anne's mother, Millie, and her father, Mike, were there, along with her sister Phyllis and her niece JoAnne. While we all sat around the kitchen table eating Anne's homegrown strawberries, I turned on the machine and we started to talk about the recipe. Anne's mother talked about how this particular dish was indigenous to the region of Italy that she was from . . . until Anne's father corrected her. Then Anne remembered how absolutely delicious it was . . . until Phyllis interrupted to tell me how important sun dried tomatoes were to the taste. Soon everybody was talking and laughing at once. That afternoon became one of those special times that friends cherish. Only when I got home and turned on the tape, the talk was so crazy and the laughter so raucous that I couldn't figure out what anyone was saying. So I had to go back a *second* time to get this recipe for you—and I promise you'll be glad I did. Enjoy!

1 teaspoon olive oil
1 teaspoon safflower oil
1 large saucepan
3 garlic cloves, minced
1 onion, diced
5 medium potatoes, peeled and diced
1 potato, peeled and cut in half
1 carrot, diced
1 celery stalk, diced
2 cups chicken broth
2 16-oz. cans cannellini beans with their liquid
½ teaspoon oregano
½ teaspoon freshly ground black pepper
sun-dried tomatoes
grated cheese

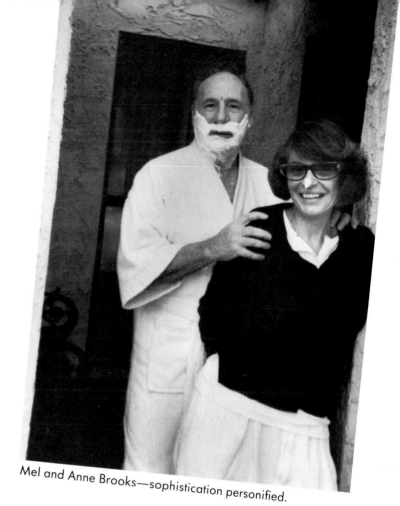

Mel and Anne Brooks—sophistication personified.

Put the oils in the saucepan and gently sauté the garlic and onion. Add all the potatoes, the carrots, celery, chicken broth, and enough water to cover the vegetables. Bring to a boil, then simmer until done (about ½ hour). Remove potato that was cut in half, mash and return to pot. Add beans, oregano, and black pepper, stir gently, and simmer for 10 minutes. Serve in soup bowls. Have some chopped sun-dried tomatoes and grated cheese on the side for those who want them.

SERVES 8–10.

ANNE BANCROFT'S VEGETARIAN CHILI

Anne Bancroft is very health-conscious; she came up with this obviously good-for-you and oh-so-delicious alternative to chili con "carne."

6   *garlic cloves, chopped fine*
2   *tablespoons olive oil*
6   *onions, coarsely chopped*
1   *cup chicken broth*
3   *medium zucchini, coarsely chopped*
2   *28-oz. cans ready-cut peeled tomatoes*
2   *12-oz. cans tomato puree*
1   *tablespoon cumin*
3   *tablespoons chili powder*
2   *teaspoons oregano*
6   *tablespoons lemon juice, or juice of 1 lemon*
½   *teaspoon cinnamon (optional)*
1   *ounce unsweetened chocolate, grated (secret)*
½   *teaspoon ground cardamom*
3   *16-oz. cans kidney beans, drained, or*
    6 cups cooked kidney beans

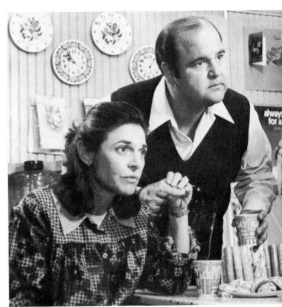

Me and Anne in a scene from *Fatso*.

In a large pot, sauté the garlic in the olive oil till golden brown, add onions and broth, and simmer over medium heat until transparent. Add zucchini. Lower heat. Add the tomatoes and tomato puree. Let simmer for a few minutes. Add cumin, chili powder, oregano, and lemon juice. Add cinnamon if you are using it. Add chocolate and cardamom. Cook 1 hour, until flavors are well blended. During last 20 minutes of cooking, add kidney beans. Serve in soup bowls.

Have separate containers of: shredded Monterey Jack cheese, shredded Cheddar cheese, chopped red onion, chopped tomato, and peeled and chopped cucumber . . . so everyone can top their own bowl of chili. Delicious with corn bread and a salad.

SERVES A BIG BUNCH!

EXTRA, EXTRA, READ ALL ABOUT IT—RED PEPPERS LIKE YOU'VE NEVER HAD THEM BEFORE!

It's traditional to cook peppers directly over a gas flame, but doing it under the broiler is equally delicious. The subtle flavor is a taste that Italians never tire of, and if you use red, green and yellow peppers, it's a colorful feast for your eyes.

6–8   large red peppers (or a combination of red, green, yellow)
2   tablespoons olive oil
1   tablespoon lemon juice
3   tablespoons capers
2   garlic cloves, whole and peeled

Preheat oven to 400 degrees.

Wash peppers and drain well.

Spread aluminum foil over the bottom of a broiling pan. Place peppers on the foil and broil until skin becomes blistered and charred. Turn peppers and do same to all sides. Remove from oven. Lift the corners of the foil and fold them together to seal in the peppers. Let stand for 30 minutes, covered with a dish towel.

Unwrap foil. Remove stems, seeds, and charred skin (which peels off very easily) from peppers, being very careful to save any and all liquid in a mixing bowl. The liquid is filled with flavor and really makes this dish.

Cut peppers into ½-inch strips and place in a mixing bowl with the reserved liquid. Add olive oil, lemon juice, capers, and garlic.

Refrigerate several hours or overnight. Great with tomatoes as an appetizer, in sandwiches, or with meat, chicken, or fish.

Note: If you push a toothpick through the whole cloves of garlic, you'll be able to find them easily, and won't eat them by mistake.

SERVES 6–8.

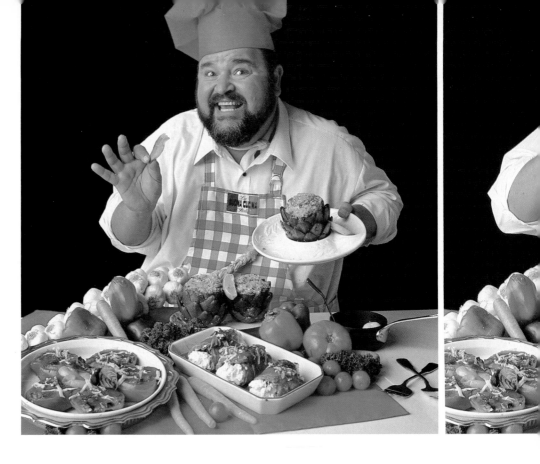

STUFFED ARTICHOKES

I once served artichokes to Randy Goodson, a friend of my son Peter's. He'd never seen an artichoke and didn't know how to eat it— but he was plucking those leaves in no time! That night we changed his name to "Randolfo Goodsono."

4   large artichokes
½   cup lemon juice
2   garlic cloves, minced
4   tablespoons olive oil
2   cups seasoned bread crumbs
2   eggs, beaten
4   tablespoons grated cheese
2   tablespoons fresh chopped parsley
    freshly ground pepper
1   cup chicken broth
    lemon wedges for garnish

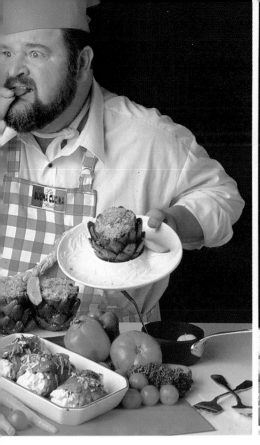
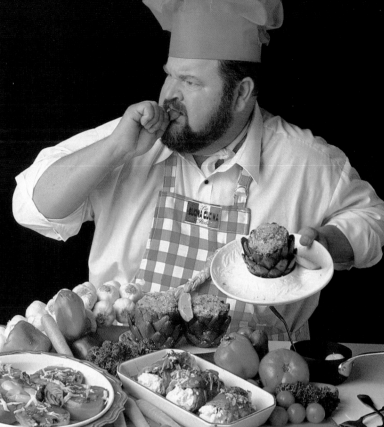

Remove the stems from the artichokes so artichokes will stand up.
Save the stems for another use. Snap off any bottom leaves that are
bruised or loose. Lay each artichoke on its side, grip firmly and cut
one inch off the top. With a scissors, trim about ¼ inch off the top of
all the leaf points. Rub artichokes with lemon juice to prevent
discoloring. Place them upside down in a large enamel kettle along
with 3 cups of water, bring to a boil, and cook for about 10 minutes.
Drain and cool. With a sharp knife, cut away the prickly tops of the
leaves. Pull out the inner core of the thistlelike leaves to expose the
choke. With a grapefruit spoon, thoroughly scrape out the hairy
choke, leaving the heart clean.

Meanwhile, in a large pan, sauté garlic in oil until golden brown.
Remove from heat. Add bread crumbs, eggs, grated cheese, parsley
and pepper. Mix together loosely. Stuff the centers of the artichokes,
and between the leaves. Place artichokes in a 9-by-12-inch baking pan.
Add the chicken broth and cover tightly with foil. Bake at 350 degrees
for 45 minutes. Remove the foil during the last 15 minutes. Serve hot
or cold with lemon wedges.

There Goes My Dinner

In all the years that Papa was working with the Department of Sanitation, he was up at 5:00 A.M., and would come home in his uniform at about 4:30 P.M. Papa loved uniforms. He treated his job with the Department of Sanitation very seriously—like a soldier. My father received "driver's" pay for twenty-five years, but he never did learn to drive a truck. When he started at the Brooklyn Sanitation Department they had horse-drawn carts, and those he knew how to drive, since he was raised on a farm. When the trucks came into use nobody bothered to change the records.

Papa was quite a man. I once saw him stop a runaway horse with his bare hands. Ralph, the vegetable man, who lived half a block from us, used a horse and wagon to travel the neighborhood selling his fresh produce. One day, when we were all sitting on our stoop, Ralph's horse was stung by a bee and went running wild down the street. My father ran right at him, grabbed his mane, pulled the horse's head down—and then bit his ear! That horse stopped dead in his tracks. I guess he was a little surprised when my father bit him. Look, let's face it—we all were. What I'm saying is, my dad was a very powerful man.

I remember one time he was yelling at us kids. The front door to our house had an upper panel of smoked glass. He often would open the door, turn, yell something at the top of his voice, then slam the door for punctuation. Usually we would all be standing there shaking with fear. I will never forget one particular time when he was into one of his tirades. He opened the door, yelled something, then slammed the door with all his might. The top glass panel broke into a thousand pieces. He just stood there, stunned. The look on his face was so hysterical that we all stopped shaking and burst out laughing!

Poor Papa. He would have these tirades, I think, because he worked so hard. But afterwards he would sheepishly sit around for days, so quiet that my heart went out to him. First he was slamming doors and breaking windows, then he was walking quietly with his hands in his pockets, shaking his head in disbelief at his own behavior.

There is a point to all of this. One of my favorite meals as a child was pasta e fagioli. Mamma served the beans and macaroni in that wonderful light tomato sauce with the garlic and olive oil with the

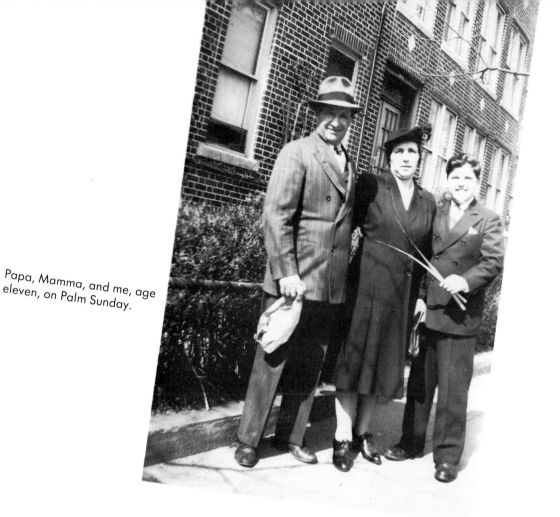

Papa, Mamma, and me, age eleven, on Palm Sunday.

fragrant grated cheese and hot crisp Italian bread . . . a little red wine . . . *two bowls!* Two bowls each before anyone spoke at the dinner table when it was pasta e fagioli night.

It was over this same glorious pasta e fagioli that I experienced something as a nine-year-old I'd like to tell you about. It wasn't the easiest thing to live through, but this story got lots of laughs in the retelling later. *Much* later.

It was dinnertime and I had my napkin tucked under my chin, and my spoon was ready, clutched in my hot little hand. My mother had just put a huge potful of pasta e fagioli in a large serving bowl. My father was all cleaned up after work. I was enjoying the feel of the fresh clean tablecloth under my hands when Mamma and Papa started to have an argument. I knew my father was tired and hungry, and I also knew that once we sat down and had some pasta e fagioli, everything was going to be all right. But it never got to the table. I guess my mother used a defiant tone and it just pushed Papa into that other dimension. Before we knew it, he had grabbed that giant serving bowl filled with my favorite pasta e fagioli and threw it up and over his shoulder so that all those beans and macaroni went flying. They seemed somehow suspended in air for one magical moment, just like a slow-motion shot in the movies. But before I knew it the pieces of broken bowl shattered on the floor, then the walls, ceiling, lamps, stove, windows—even the curtains—were covered with pasta e fagioli! My father jerked open the door to the apartment screaming, "I no see no ting like this my whole life!" He slammed the door behind him.

I thought, I never saw anything like this in my whole life either, Pop.

I can see myself sitting there with my napkin still tucked under my chin, the spoon still in my hand, with nothing to eat. The whole family was stunned. After a while we cleaned up the kitchen as best we could. I was scared at first, but then I got silly and started to imitate Papa. I took a dish towel and shaped it into a fake bowl, then threw the dish towel into the air—just as he walked into the kitchen. We froze. Papa looked around and then quietly walked into the living room.

Months later, when I was changing a light bulb in the kitchen, I found a bean and a macaroni stuck to the ceiling to remind me of that evening. "Wow!" I thought. "He got it way up here?" Shortly after that I noticed our picture of St. Theresa—and she had a wart! But of course it was only an old dry bean from Papa's passion. For years, especially during spring cleaning, we kept finding them. When Papa was angry, he was angry.

Nowadays beans and macaroni is still one of my favorite dishes, but I never eat it without thinking back on that night in Brooklyn when we were visited by the "Fabulous Flying Pasta Fagiolis."

MAMMA'S PASTA E FAGIOLI

2 *garlic cloves, minced*
2 *tablespoons olive oil*
1 *8-oz. can tomato sauce*
1 *cup water*
1 *16-oz. can cannellini beans*
½ *pound of ditalini or elbow macaroni*
  fresh parsley, chopped
  grated cheese

In a saucepan, fry the garlic gently in the oil until golden brown. Add the tomato sauce and water, and let cook 10 minutes. Add beans, stir gently, continue to cook on simmer.

Cook ditalini or elbow macaroni al dente, drain, and add to bean mixture. Stir gently. If it gets too thick, add a little more water. Add parsley.

Serve immediately, or else the pasta will absorb all the liquid. This is so good that I would double the recipe, because it is delicious when sprinkled with grated cheese, with Italian bread dipped in the sauce. Some people love it cold the next day, or you can add a little water and warm it up.

Enjoy!

SERVES 4.

Variations: Omit the can of tomato sauce and it becomes a "white sauce" utilizing the white bean juice.

Pasta e fagioli is great with a sprinkle of crushed, dried hot pepper flakes.

Alternative: Replace cannellini beans with a can of chick peas, sweet peas, blackeye peas, or lima beans . . . whatever matches your wallpaper best!

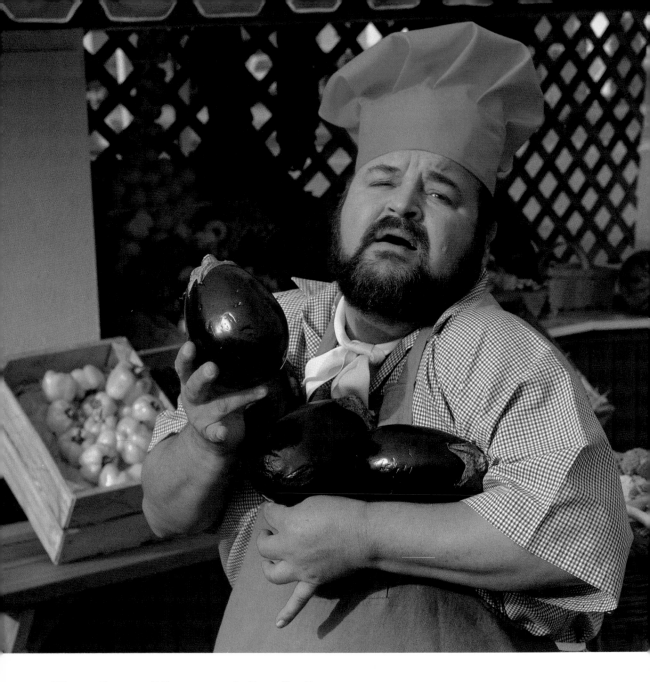

Eggplant: Nectar of the Gods

Eggplant is to an Italian what sex is to a nymphomaniac. You *can* exist, but without it what's the use of living?

There are a lot of things you can do with eggplants, and here are some of them. Have fun!

DOM'S MOM'S STUFFED EGGPLANT ROLLS

This creation of Mamma's is one of my personal favorites. It's healthy, it looks fabulous, and it's delicious with meat and/or a side dish of pasta.

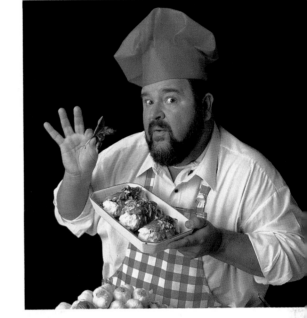

2   *medium eggplants*
    flour for dredging
2   *eggs, beaten*
    olive oil
½   *pound sliced mozzarella*
1   *pound ricotta mixed with 1 tablespoon of finely chopped parsley*
2   *cups Mamma's Marinara Sauce (page 120)*
    more chopped parsley, if desired
    grated cheese, if desired

Wash eggplants, remove stems, peel, and slice lengthwise. Dredge eggplant slices in flour. Dip into beaten egg and fry until golden brown. Pat dry with paper towels. Place a slice of mozzarella in the middle of each eggplant slice. Add a scoop of ricotta. Roll up eggplant slices and place eggplant rolls, seam side down, in greased shallow baking pan and top with a little Marinara Sauce.

Bake in a 350-degree oven for 15 to 30 minutes. If desired, garnish with chopped parsley, and grated cheese. Great with a pasta on the side!

SERVES 8–10.

EGGPLANT-STUFFED PEPPERS

When Sal Sicari, my musical conductor/arranger, and I travel around the country, we end up eating in a lot of coffee shops and so we *long* for some home-cooked food. Once when we got back to Brooklyn, New York, Sal's wife, Geri, a wiz in the kitchen, came to the rescue with this vegetarian delight. I begged her for the recipe and here it is:

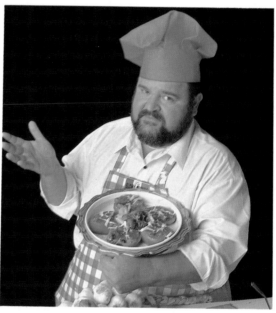

1   *large eggplant, peeled and
    cut into bite-size pieces*
2   *tablespoons oil*
3   *garlic cloves, minced*
1   *cup flavored bread crumbs*
½   *cup (or more) fresh basil, chopped fine*
½   *cup (or more) grated cheese*
½   *pound mozzarella, sliced
    pepper to taste*
½   *cup fresh parsley*
4   *red bell peppers, cut in half lengthwise,
    seeded and pith removed, and parboiled
    Mamma's Marinara Sauce (page 120)*

Sauté pieces of eggplant in the oil, with the minced garlic, until the eggplant is very soft (about 30 minutes). Stir in the bread crumbs until all are moistened. Sprinkle with fresh basil (about 6 leaves, chopped fine). Add the grated cheese, pepper and parsley.

Fill parboiled peppers halfway with the eggplant mixture, then put a slice of mozzarella in each center and cover with more of the eggplant mixture.

Place in baking pan with ½ cup of water and bake at 350 degrees for 1 hour. Sprinkle top with a little more fresh basil and more grated cheese and top with Mamma's Marinara Sauce.

I am telling you, no one will know that this incredibly subtle, delicious vegetable filling is eggplant.

SERVES 4–6.

DOM'S RATATOUILLE

I gave this recipe to my sister Anne. She made it and said all her guests flipped over it. We both agree it is the best ratatouille in the whole world, and folks, it can have okra in it, which is a great vegetable that a lot of people don't even know about! P.S. Even if you choose to omit okra, you'll still have the best-tasting ratatouille in the whole world anyway.

4	*tablespoons olive oil*
3	*garlic cloves, peeled and chopped fine*
1	*onion, chopped*
2	*zucchini, sliced*
1	*eggplant, peeled and cubed*
2	*celery stalks, sliced*
4	*okra pods, sliced (optional)*
2	*carrots, sliced*
1	*green pepper, sliced*
1	*red pepper, sliced*
8–10	*mushrooms, sliced*
3	*tablespoons flour*
5	*ripe tomatoes, peeled and sliced, or 1 28-oz. can crushed tomatoes*
	freshly ground black pepper to taste
4	*teaspoons chopped fresh parsley*
1	*teaspoon oregano*
1	*teaspoon basil*

In a large skillet, heat olive oil and sauté garlic and onions. Lightly flour remaining vegetables, except tomatoes, and add to skillet along with tomatoes, pepper, parsley, oregano and basil. Cook over medium flame for 30 minutes. Stir, lower flame, and then simmer for 1 hour.

Delicious hot or cold as a vegetable, or great at a summer buffet.

SERVES 8–10.

RITA'S RECIPE FROM FELINA IN ITALY
(Open-faced eggplant sandwich)

My sister-in-law is a tall, redheaded lady who makes wonderful children—and some delicious dishes too! She swears by this one.

1 large eggplant, unpeeled and chopped
2 medium peppers, chopped
2 large garlic cloves, minced
2 tablespoons olive oil
1 loaf Italian bread
1 chopped tomato
1 small head escarole, chopped and steamed a bit
   wine vinegar
   capers
   black olives, sliced
   fresh basil

Gently fry the eggplant and peppers with the crushed garlic in the olive oil about 15 minutes.

Cut the bread in half lengthwise and divide the eggplant, peppers, tomatoes, and escarole between each half. Place in oven and bake at 300 degrees for 15–20 minutes.

Sprinkle with wine vinegar, capers, olives, and basil. Serve on a warm platter. It's very Italian and it's surprisingly delicious.

SERVES 4.

FATHER ORSINI'S EGGPLANT BALLS

Some time ago, I co-hosted the Mike Douglas show in Philadelphia for a week and got a chance to fulfill some fantasies! I sang, philosophized, cooked with my mother, danced with Ginger Rogers, and rode on the back of a wild ostrich. I loved it! Mike and his lovely wife, Gen, were extremely kind to Carol and me, and I cherish their friendship. . . .

During that week, one of the guests was Father Joseph Orsini, a warm-hearted priest who had grown up in the streets of Bayonne,

New Jersey, and had written a cookbook called *Papa Bear's Favorite Italian Dishes*. (Orsini comes from *orso*—Italian for bear.) On the show, Father Orsini made, excuse the expression, eggplant balls that can be used in an antipasto or in place of meatballs on spaghetti. Despite my Italian upbringing, I had never heard about eggplant balls, but have cooked them happily many times since. I'm also proud to call Father Orsini my friend. Bless me, Father, I could use it!

3   tablespoons olive oil
3   garlic cloves, minced
1   large eggplant, peeled and diced
1   tablespoon water
1   cup seasoned bread crumbs
½   cup fresh parsley, chopped
2   eggs, beaten
½   cup grated cheese
     olive oil
     marinara sauce, if desired
     grated mozzarella or
Monterey Jack, if desired

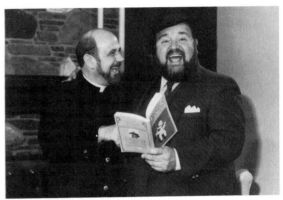

Me and Father Orsini laughing at life.

In a large saucepan, heat oil and gently sauté garlic until golden brown. Add diced eggplant, the tablespoon of water, and cover. Reduce heat and gently steam until eggplant is *very soft*.

In a mixing bowl, combine eggplant, bread crumbs, parsley, eggs, and cheese. Mix well and let stand 20 minutes. Form into balls and fry on all sides in olive oil.

or:

Place eggplant balls on a greased pan, and bake in the oven for 30 minutes at 325 degrees. They can be covered with marinara sauce and sprinkled with grated mozzarella or Monterey Jack.

or:

Drop them in spaghetti sauce and serve in place of meatballs.
Thanks, Father!

SERVES 4–6.

Note: A special thanks to Logos International, Plainfield, New Jersey, for permission to use this recipe.

Here are three stuffed mushroom recipes representing the DeLuise family. You may be wondering why my mother, my sister and I all have different recipes for stuffed mushrooms. Our recipes started out the same, but since all of us cook, each of us went off in a different direction and so did our mushrooms! They're all delicious, although modesty forbids me to tell you which I prefer. This first recipe is a wonderful accompaniment to an almost all-vegetable dinner, because it uses very little meat. These mushrooms also make great hors d'oeuvres, and go well with a primavera on the side.

MAMMA'S STUFFED MUSHROOMS

2 garlic cloves, minced
1 teaspoon olive oil
2 sweet Italian sausages
5 tablespoons flavored bread crumbs
1 teaspoon grated cheese

1 tablespoon minced parsley
1 egg
1 pound mushrooms
   chicken stock

In a frying pan, gently brown the minced garlic in the olive oil. Remove the sausage meat from the casing, crumble the meat into the pan, and brown that, too. In a bowl, combine the bread crumbs, cheese, parsley, and egg. Add the cooked sausage.

Wash the mushrooms quickly, because they tend to absorb water. Remove the mushroom stems and save them for soup, or mince them and put them back into the stuffing. Fill the caps nicely with the stuffing. Place them in a baking pan lined with foil. Add a little chicken stock to the bottom of the pan (6–10 tablespoons), just to give them moisture.

Bake at 325 degrees for 30 minutes. If the mushrooms are small, maybe 15 minutes will do. Serve them hot!

SERVES 4–6.

DOM'S STUFFED MUSHROOMS

I serve these mushrooms with a main course, but I feel they are best when used in a buffet.

1	*pound medium-size mushrooms*	*1*	*cup seasoned bread crumbs*
1	*small onion, finely chopped*	*½*	*cup grated Parmesan cheese*
2	*garlic cloves, minced*	*2*	*teaspoons parsley*
2–3	*tablespoons olive oil*	*2*	*teaspoons soy sauce*
1	*egg, beaten*	*4*	*tablespoons water*

Wash mushrooms, remove stems, and set caps aside. Brown onions and garlic in olive oil. Finely chop mushroom stems, add to onion and garlic, and brown over low heat.

Combine onions, mushroom stems, egg, bread crumbs, cheese, and parsley in a bowl and mix. Stuff mushroom caps with mixture.

Place mushrooms in a baking dish with soy sauce and water on the bottom. Cover with foil and bake at 350 degrees for 10 minutes. Uncover and continue baking until tops are golden brown. Serve hot to accompany broiled or roasted meat, or as an appetizer.

SERVES 4–6.

MY SISTER ANNE'S STUFFED MUSHROOMS

Accompany this recipe with a simple green salad, and you've created what looks like the perfect light lunch to me!

2	*pounds large mushrooms*	*1½*	*cups seasoned bread crumbs*
2	*tablespoons olive oil*	*2*	*cups crab meat*
2	*garlic cloves, minced*		*pepper to taste*
1	*onion, minced*	*1*	*cup Monterey Jack cheese, shredded*

Wash mushrooms quickly and remove stems. Mince stems and set mushrooms aside.

Heat oil in a skillet and sauté garlic, onion, 1 cup of seasoned bread crumbs, and the minced mushroom stems. Remove from heat, add crab meat and sprinkle with pepper. Mix together well.

Stuff mushrom caps with mixture. Place in a casserole dish and top with remaining bread crumbs and the grated cheese. Bake at 350 degrees for 20 minutes.

SERVES 6–8.

MAMMA'S SPINACH ROLLS

When anybody is working with flour and dough, it's always fascinating to children. I remember when I was a little kid, with my nose just above the counter, I used to love to watch my mother lovingly roll out the dough. Then Mamma would let me climb on a chair so I could roll out my own. I remember how proud and excited I was when *my* spinach roll came out of the oven. I recently taught my seventeen-year-old son, Michael, how to make this, and I guess he wasn't too old to get into this terrific dish because he ate the whole thing for dinner!

> *Pizza Dough (page 207)*
> 1 *pound fresh spinach, washed, drained, and coarsely chopped*
> 1 *small onion, chopped*
>   *grated cheese*
>   *pinch of red pepper*
>   *olive oil*
> 1 *egg, beaten*

Roll out pizza dough into a thin rectangle and place on greased cookie sheet. Spread chopped spinach evenly over dough. Sprinkle with chopped onion, cheese and pepper. Drizzle olive oil over, then gently roll dough jellyroll fashion, making sure the seam is on the bottom. Shape into a crescent.

Using a fork, poke 8–10 holes in the dough so it can "breathe," and brush roll with beaten egg. Bake at 350 degrees for 40 minutes. Slice and serve hot or cold as an appetizer, or with a salad, for a delicious, healthful light meal.

SERVES 4–6.

Variation: Substitute 2 cups chopped broccoli and 1 cup of shredded mozzarella for spinach.

EVERYBODY'S POT LE GEL

Carl Reiner and Jack Gilford are both great friends of mine and have a lot of things in common. They are both very funny men. Both live in Los Angeles . . . except Jack, who lives in New York. Both have a wife named Estelle who sings . . . except for Jack . . . whose wife's name is Madeline who is a producer. Both have two boys and a girl, and one of the sons is named Rob, who is an actor/director . . . except for Jack . . . who has two boys and a girl, and one of his sons is named Joe, who is a director. Whew! Both will always bring Pot le Gel (the Romanian word for eggplant) to a potluck supper, and both call it Carl's mother's recipe for Pot le Gel . . . except for Jack . . . who calls it Jack's mother's recipe for Pot le Gel. Just know that whatever *you* choose to call it, it's fantastic!

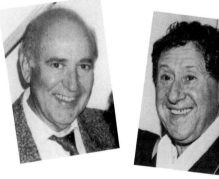

1 *eggplant*
   juice of 1 lemon
3 *tablespoons olive oil*
   salt
   pepper
1 *onion, minced*
1 *tomato, chopped*

Over a very low gas flame, place the eggplant directly on the burner for about 15 minutes or until eggplant chars, and then turn and char the other side for 20 minutes. If you have an electric stove, do this step under the broiler. Eggplant will get black, ooze and drip. On a drainboard that slants toward the sink, remove the pulp with a wooden spoon and discard the skin. Squeeze out all the excess juice and put the pulp in a mixing bowl. Squeeze in the lemon juice, which gives the eggplant a good flavor and also keeps it white. Add the olive oil, salt, pepper, minced onion and chopped tomato and mix together. Serve in a bowl with crackers.

Note: This is often referred to as the "Poor Man's Caviar." Thank you so much, Carl. And you too, Jack.

SERVES 4–6.

Pasta, Sauces, Rice, and Other Grains

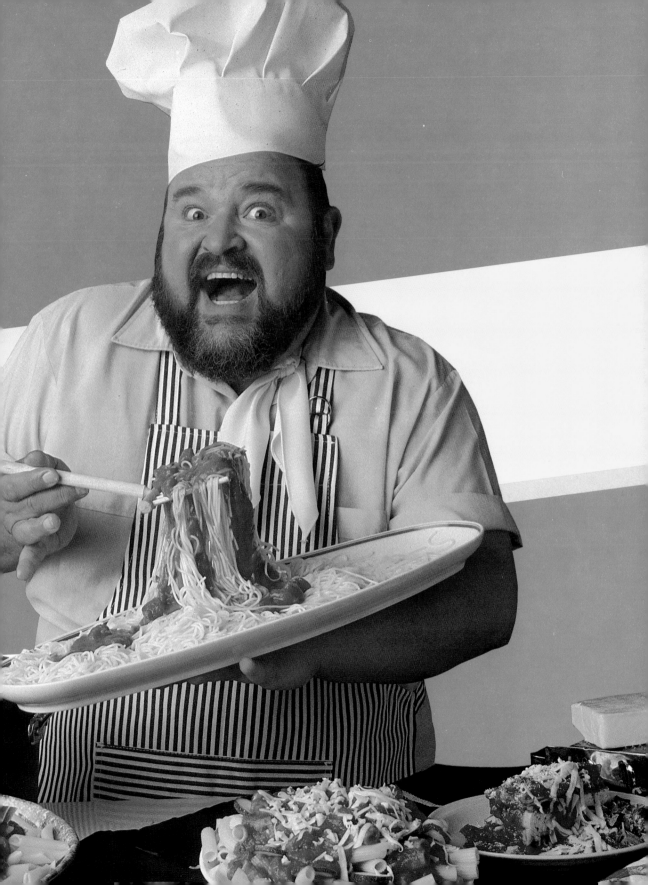

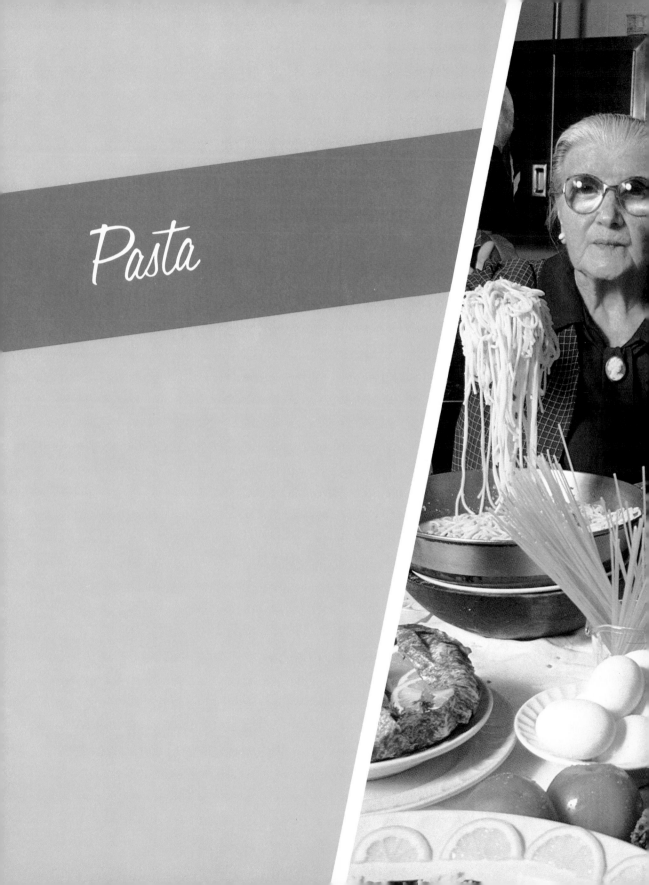

Pasta

This memory is as vivid to me as my first kiss. I am about eight years old, lying in my bed with my face in the pillow: one eye opens quickly as the aroma of garlic and tomato sauce makes its way to my bedroom. I sit up, smile, jump into my old blue bathrobe, wander into the kitchen and see that my mother has prepared for "surgery." She's wearing a large white apron over her housedress, and a thin white towel has been wrapped around her head so that no hair is visible. She looks like Florence Nightingale in her finest hour. Her hands are covered with flour, she's standing in front of a large piece of wood that's been placed over our kitchen table, and she's making my favorite pasta of all: "Homemade Macs." She gives me a kiss and says, "Good morning, sleepyhead."

Now, I also want to tell you that my mother, like all the mothers in our neighborhood, also made tomato sauce every Sunday morning, and that spaghetti sauce was cooking for at least an hour before anyone else in the family got up. So by the time I came downstairs, I knew the sauce was ready for tasting. I took a slice of Italian bread and put a little tomato sauce on it, then sprinkled it with grated

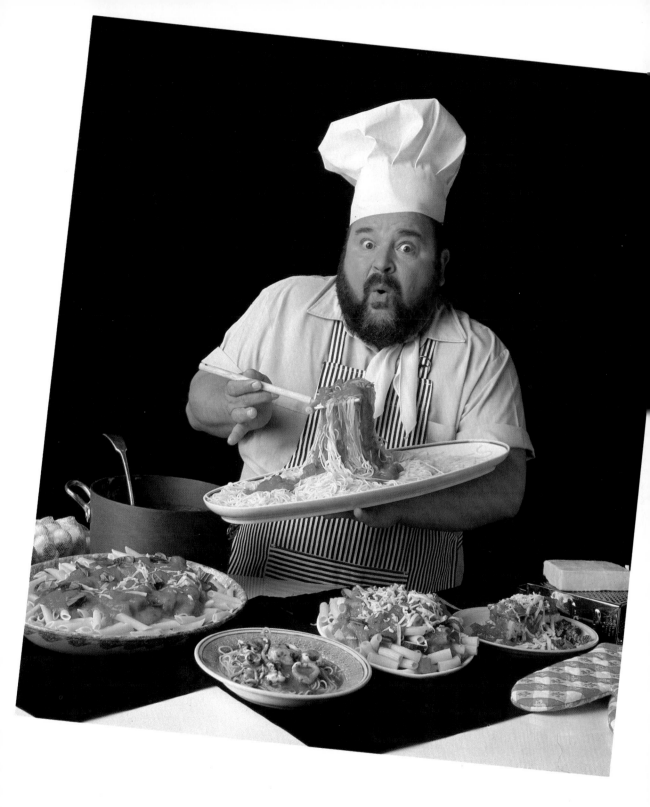

cheese. I *really* loved this Sunday ritual. Then I sat in the kitchen and watched her happily make pasta for at least eight people. The problem of drying it was solved by putting clean sheets on top of the bedspread and on bureaus, tables, anything that was flat. This process took hours. Even *longer* if she made ravioli. By the time Mamma was finished laying out the pasta to dry, our house looked like a hospital for wounded spaghetti! Finally she shooed me off to get dressed while she put on her black dress, little pearl earrings and hat for church. During the mass, God forgive me, all I thought about was pasta, pasta, pasta!

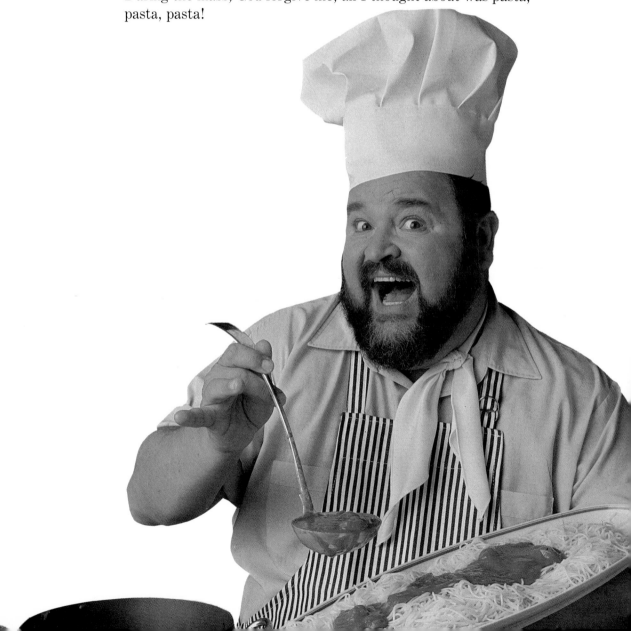

FRESH PASTA

I ask many of my friends this hypothetical question: If they were on a desert island with only one food to live on, what *one* food would they choose? Some say soup, some say nuts, but Carl Reiner, Mel Brooks, Anne Bancroft, Charles Nelson Reilly, Vic Damone, Dean Martin, Frank Sinatra, Luciano Pavarotti, and me all say "Pasta!" Al dente, of course. (Al dente means that you cook the pasta only until it is just tender but still resistant to your bite.)

Don't be afraid of making your own pasta. Give it a chance. I bet you'll find it's much easier than you think, therapeutic, and really a lot of fun. Fresh pasta! It's a thrill to create, and oh so satisfying when you and your guests taste the difference.

3 cups semolina flour
2 tablespoons olive oil
1 cup warm water

Put flour onto board, make a center well, add olive oil, and a small amount of water. Mix, bringing flour from around edges, kneading together. Add more water, if needed; continue kneading until dough will form a smooth ball. Cover dough with a bowl and let it rest for 10 minutes. Re-knead until dough is smooth. Cover again with bowl for 15 minutes, then divide dough ball into 3 pieces and roll into ⅛-inch sheets. Cut strips into desired widths, or use small pasta machine that has dies for making fresh spaghetti or other forms. Dry for 1 hour before cooking.

Fresh pasta cooks much more quickly than dry.

SERVES 4–5.

EGG PASTA FOR RAVIOLI OR MANICOTTI

4 cups semolina flour
3 large eggs, lightly beaten
1 tablespoon olive oil
2 tablespoons warm water

Put flour onto board. Make a center well, add the eggs and oil. Gradually mix well, kneading into a soft, smooth dough. Knead from 5 to 10 minutes, long enough to have a smooth, elastic dough; cover with pan or bowl for ½ hour.

SERVES 6–8, USED AS RAVIOLI OR MANICOTTI.

SPINACH PASTA

1 pound fresh spinach, well washed
4 cups semolina flour
2 eggs, lightly beaten

In a saucepan, steam spinach in 4 tablespoons water, well covered, until tender. Drain well, pressing out all the water. Then force through a food mill, or chop in a food processor.

Put the flour onto a board, make a center well and add the beaten eggs, and finally the spinach. Now knead until the dough is well mixed. Knead for 15 minutes, until it is smooth, adding water if it is too dry or flour if too soft.

Makes a healthy pound!

SERVES 5–6.

Gnocchi: The Italian Dumpling

I think you'll find these to be absolutely wonderful . . . they are much lighter than the traditional gnocchi. *Please* try them!

GNOCCHI #1

2 cups flour
2 cups ricotta cheese
2 eggs

Put flour, ricotta, and eggs in mixing bowl, and with a large spoon blend ingredients into a large ball. Place dough on a floured board and roll into a ball again. Add more flour, if necessary, to prevent sticking. Roll small amounts of dough, forming cigar-sized strands. Cut each strand into 1-inch pieces. With your knuckle or index finger, form a dent in the center of each.

Drop into lots of boiling water (they will sink) and cook about 8–10 minutes. When the gnocchi float to the top of the boiling water they are done.

Drain and place on a large platter. Top with Mamma's Marinara Sauce (page 120), grated cheese, and coarsely chopped fresh basil.

SERVES 4–8.

GNOCCHI #2

3   medium potatoes
2   eggs
1¼ cups flour

Peel, cut and boil potatoes until you can pierce them easily with a fork, but don't overcook. Drain and put in a mixing bowl. Add the eggs and whip until fluffy. Add the flour. Turn onto a floured board and knead dough with the hands till smooth, adding more flour, if necessary, to prevent sticking and forming into a bowl.

Take a small handful of dough and with your hands roll it out into a long rope. Cut the rope into inch-long pieces, and then flatten each piece slightly. With knuckle of your index finger, gently dent the center of each piece. Drop into lots of boiling water and cook for 8–10 minutes. When they float, they are ready. Drain and place on platter.

Serve with your favorite spaghetti sauce and grated cheese, and sprinkle fresh basil on top.

SERVES 6–8.

GNOCCHI VERDI

This is festive, light, and "green." Who could ask for anything more!

1	pound spinach
2	cups ricotta cheese
1½	cups grated cheese
3	eggs
¼	teaspoon nutmeg
4	tablespoons parsley, finely minced
	grated rind of 1 lemon
1	cup flour
	pepper to taste
8	tablespoons butter, melted
	chopped fresh basil

Wash spinach. Steam and drain well, pressing out any excess water. Puree spinach in a food processor and add the ricotta, 1 cup of the grated cheese, the eggs, nutmeg, parsley, lemon rind, flour, and pepper. Process until well blended. (If you don't have a food processor, steam as above, chop the spinach fine, put it in a large mixing bowl with the rest of the ingredients above, and mix thoroughly. Then continue as below.)

Remove from bowl of processor (or from mixing bowl), turn out onto a floured board, and form into a smooth ball, adding small amounts of flour, if necessary.

Form and cook the gnocchi according to instructions on page 105. Drain well, turn into a warmed bowl, toss gently with the melted butter, sprinkle with basil, and serve immediately, passing the remaining grated cheese at the table.

SERVES 6.

P.S. Or try them with your favorite sauce.

BROCCOLI WITH RIGATONI

Without a doubt, here is a combination made in *heaven!*

8 *tablespoons olive oil*
2 *tablespoons butter*
4 *garlic cloves, minced*
1 *bunch broccoli, separated into florets (reserve stems for another use)*
1 *cup chicken broth*
1 *cup fresh basil, coarsely chopped*
1 *pound rigatoni*
  fresh parsley, chopped
  pepper
  grated cheese

In a large skillet, heat oil and butter and gently brown the garlic. Add broccoli and stir gently until pan gets very hot. Add chicken broth, cover, and simmer just until broccoli is al dente.

Add half the fresh basil and the drained hot rigatoni, cooked al dente, to the skillet and mix thoroughly. Put on a hot serving dish and sprinkle with parsley, pepper, grated cheese, and remaining basil.

Fabulous! Serve with a tossed green salad.

SERVES 4.

I also like fusilli for this dish just as well.

LUCY'S PASTA

The DePaolos had the apartment upstairs from us in Brooklyn when I was fifteen years old. Lucy (Mrs. DePaolo) was like a second mother to me. Since she came from a different region (Naples) than my parents, she would make different pastas than Mamma. One day I tasted this incredible new dish, and decided to get Lucy's recipe. Recently I made it for my three sons, who carried me around on their shoulders after dinner! This is a no-meat, no-tomato sauce, and if you want to taste a very "easy to get hooked on" pasta—this is it! Thanks, Mom #2.

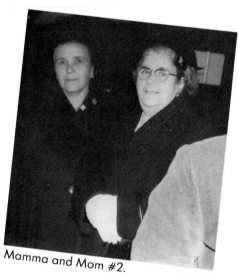

Mamma and Mom #2.

5	fresh garlic cloves, minced
⅓	cup olive oil
3	onions, sliced into thin crescents
½	cup fresh parsley, finely chopped
1	pound spaghetti or linguine
3 or 4	large eggs
4	tablespoons grated cheese
½	cup fresh basil torn into small pieces
	freshly ground pepper to taste
	additional fresh, coarsely chopped parsley, basil, and grated cheese to taste

Brown garlic in olive oil. Add onions and gently sauté until onions are crunchy and brown. When onions are almost done, add the ½ cup parsley and sauté gently until limp.

Cook pasta in boiling water until al dente. While pasta is cooking, beat together eggs, cheese, and the ½ cup of basil. Drain and place hot pasta in a serving bowl and fold in the egg mixture (the heat from the pasta will cook the eggs). Add contents of frying pan and mix well. Sprinkle with pepper and serve with more fresh parsley, basil, and grated cheese, as desired. This combination is so tasty and unique, I feel you'll thank me, even though I ain't there to enjoy it with you.

SERVES 4–6.

DOM'S PRIMAVERA

My wife, Carol, can and *does* live on this dish.

5	garlic cloves, *minced*
4	tablespoons olive oil
2	tablespoons butter
½	pound asparagus, *cut in bite-sized pieces*
2	zucchini, *thinly sliced*
2	carrots, *thinly sliced*
½	cup peas
1	cup broccoli *florets*
1	cup cauliflower *florets*
1	onion, *sliced in crescents*
6	leaves of fresh basil, *chopped*
1	cup chicken broth
8–10	mushrooms, *sliced*
1	pound rigatoni *grated cheese*

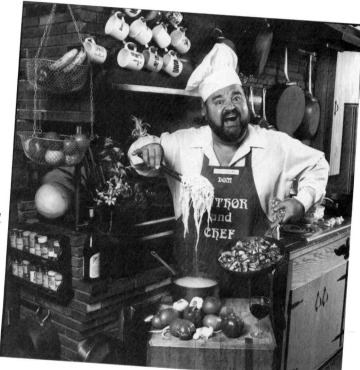

In a large skillet, sauté garlic in oil. Add vegetables and basil and sauté until almost tender. Add chicken broth and mushrooms. Bring to a boil, quickly reduce heat, cover, and simmer for 5 minutes. Mix well. Serve over pasta cooked al dente. Sprinkle with grated cheese.

SERVES 6.

Variation #1: When adding chicken broth, first mix well with 1 can of cream of mushroom soup (it works!).

Variation #2: Omit chicken broth. Instead, add 1 28-oz. can of ready-cut or crushed tomatoes.

Variation #3: 1 cup of diced cooked chicken may be added when you add the chicken broth.

PESTO ALLA BATTISTA

Carol and I have an actor friend, Lloyd Battista, who has an uncanny ability to pick out varied, unique, and inexpensive restaurants that serve the most delicious food our family has tasted. Our boys are real impressed with his ability. Lloyd has a mellow baritone voice and an imposing great nose. Always, when the DeLuises all agree that Lloyd has discovered for us yet another fabulous restaurant, our sweet friend will point to the front of his face and say in his booming voice, "The nose knows!" Lloyd introduced our family to this untraditional pesto sauce. When I suggested a change in the recipe, my three sons sang out, "Dad, you can't! The nose knows!"

⅓	*cup olive oil*
1	*cup (or more) fresh basil leaves*
1	*cup pine nuts*
3 or 4	*cloves garlic*
⅓	*cup grated cheese*
	pepper
1	*pound ripe tomatoes, peeled*
	or
1	*28-oz. can ready-cut tomatoes*
1	*pound linguine or fettuccine*

Pour the olive oil into a blender and add the basil, ½ cup of the pine nuts and garlic and blend until it's a smooth paste. Pour mixture into a bowl and add the grated cheese and pepper. Mix well.

Put a strainer over the bowl and, if you are using the fresh tomatoes, cut them in half over it so the juice goes in the bowl. Scoop out the seeds into the strainer and squash all the juice and pulp adhering to them into the bowl. Discard the seeds.

If using canned tomatoes, skip the strainer, chop the tomatoes into the pesto, and use only ¾ of the juice from the can. Stir to blend.

Leave sauce out at room temperature—*don't heat or cook.*

Cook pasta and drain well. Pour sauce over pasta and sprinkle with grated cheese and the remaining ½ cup of pine nuts.

SERVES 4–6.

Shut Up and Eat Your Lasagne

When Carol and I were engaged to be married, she came to Brooklyn to "meet the family." As you can imagine, they were excited to meet her because I told them that I was very serious about this girl from East Rutherford, New Jersey, whose father was a cop, and who was in show business. I also told them they should all go easy on her. So my mother fixed one of her incredible dinners from soup to nuts and everything in between. When she brought out the antipasto, there were ooohs and aaahs . . . after we tasted her incredible lasagne, there was applause, whistles and cheers. Mamma even stood up and took a bow! Everyone was on their best behavior. Papa sat at the head of the table, and he was wearing a tie. I mean, I have to tell you, that was something! My brother Nick was there, and his wife, Rita, and their four kids, Candida, Dolores, John, Regina, my sister Anne, my brother-in-law Phil, who used to be a fighter in the Golden Gloves, their children, Concetta, John, and Mary, my mother, me, and, of course, the soon-to-be-my-wife, Carol. When I say my family was on their best behavior, I mean *best behavior*. Not one meatball was thrown! My brother-in-law Phil was sitting next to me and in the middle of dinner, I asked him what he thought of Carol, who had just finished her lasagne. He looked at her, smiled at me and said, "She's got a terrific appetite!" Just then, Papa took his spoon and tapped his wine glass and said, "I wanna aska Carol a question." Everyone became quiet. Now Papa spoke very broken English and he said, "If is be one fruits, inna da wholes worls, which is be the best fruits for the mans?"

I quickly translated and said, "Carol, my father wants to know if you had to pick one fruit in the whole wide world, what would be the best fruit for a man to pick?"

Everyone stopped eating, forks were placed quietly on the tablecloth, all heads slowly turned toward Carol, she looked around, realizing that this was a very important moment in our relationship, took a deep breath, let out a sigh, and said, "An orange."

There was what seemed to be an endless pause . . . until my father pounded the table and proclaimed, "She's a right!" Everyone relaxed. Papa winked at Carol. There was a burst of applause and cheering that lasted for two minutes.

Then it was Carol's turn to take a bow. She had passed the "fruit test." Papa explained that it was nourishing, and it had juice and was, I guess, his favorite fruit. To this day, Carol doesn't know why she said orange. Wasn't it lucky that she said orange . . . I mean, so that I could marry her, you know? What if she'd said apple? Anyway, I leaned toward Carol and said, "Orange you glad you came?" Carol smiled and said, "Shut up and eat your lasagne."

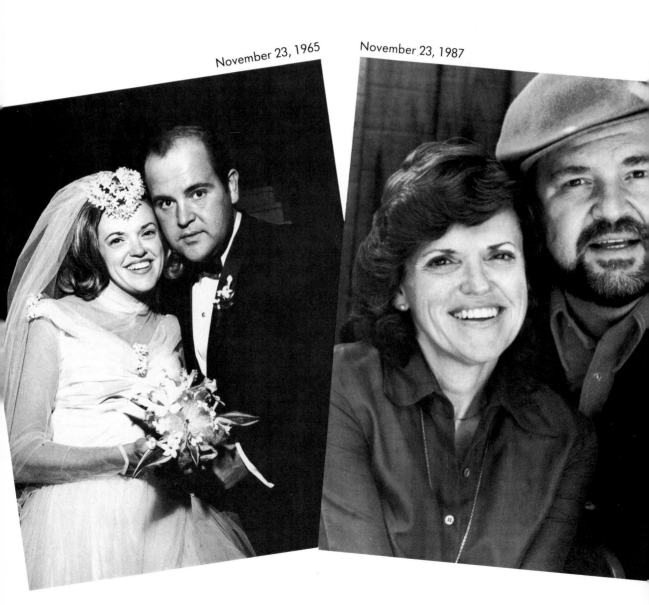

November 23, 1965

November 23, 1987

LASAGNE

1 *pound lasagne noodles*
2 *quarts Mamma's Marinara Sauce (page 120)*
   or sauce of your choice
2 *pounds ricotta cheese*
1 *pound mozzarella cheese*
1 *cup grated Parmesan cheese*

Cook lasagne noodles al dente. Drain. Preheat oven to 325 degrees.

Using a baking dish about 2½ inches deep, cover the bottom with sauce of your choice and line the dish with a layer of lasagne. Dot with spoonfuls of ricotta, slices of mozzarella and some grated Parmesan cheese. Cover with sauce. Repeat with another layer of lasagne, sauce, and cheeses, until baking dish is almost filled.

Bake about 45 minutes. Cool 20 minutes before serving.

Serve with additional sauce.

SERVES 8–10.

Optional: You can add slices of cooked sausage or small meatballs to each layer.

Dom's Note: When you just don't have time to prepare this dish and you want it yesterday, do what I do: I simply start with a deep lasagne pan and all cold ingredients. Start with ½ cup of the sauce and use raw, uncooked lasagne noodles, one layer of ricotta, mozzarella, and grated cheese, then sauce . . . another layer of raw, uncooked lasagne noodles at right angles to the first, and so on, and so on. You finish with the sauce.

Cover with aluminum foil very snug around the top, place in a 350-degree oven and bake for 1½ hours. Let stand 20 minutes. This can be done ahead. It cuts beautifully and you can reheat and serve pieces in individual baking dishes with additional sauce.

Try it, you'll like it!

MA ZITI'S STUFFED SHELLS

When I married Carol, I got a mother-in-law named Mildred, I got a brother-in-law named George, and I got a sister-in-law named "Ma Ziti." Her real name is Midge, and we're very much alike. She minces garlic with one hand tied behind her back! The first time I went to Ma Ziti's house for dinner, there were two soups, four entrees, three frittatas and twelve desserts. Ma Ziti is beautiful and energetic, and if she's not cooking gallons of spaghetti sauce, making strawberry jam, or pickling watermelon rinds, she's sleeping. Of course, on special occasions, she has been known to make ziti. Baked ziti . . . and now you know how she got her nickname. Midge is a fine chef. She learned to cook from her dad, and she graduated "Pasta Cum Laude." This is how Ma Ziti stuffs her shells:

2   quarts *Mamma's Marinara* or *Meat Sauce* (see under *Sauces*)
2   eggs
1   pound ricotta cheese
½   pound mozzarella cheese, grated
½   cup grated Parmesan cheese
4   tablespoons parsley
    few leaves of basil, chopped
    dash of pepper
24 giant ziti shells
    grated cheese for the top

Make Mamma's sauce (whichever one you decide on) and set aside.

In a large bowl, combine the eggs, ricotta, mozzarella and Parmesan cheeses, parsley, basil, and pepper.

Cook giant shells in lots of boiling water until al dente. Careful! Don't overcook. If they are too limp, it's harder to fill these suckers. Drain, and stuff each shell with a few tablespoons of the cheese mixture.

Cover the bottom of a large baking dish with about ½ inch of Mamma's sauce. Arrange stuffed shells side by side in the sauce. Dribble the remaining sauce over the top and down the center of the shells. Sprinkle the additional Parmesan cheese over the top and bake, covered, in a 350-degree oven until hot and bubbly.

Delicious with a green salad and hot, crusty bread.

Variations:

1. Sauté 1 minced garlic clove and 1 finely chopped onion in a bit of oil until golden brown. Add 1 package (10 ounces) of frozen chopped spinach, thawed and well drained; cook briefly with garlic and onion and combine with the cheese mixture. Add sauce as above.

2. Sauté 1 pound of lean ground beef or veal, 1 minced garlic clove and 1 finely chopped onion and add to cheese mixture.

SERVES 6–8.

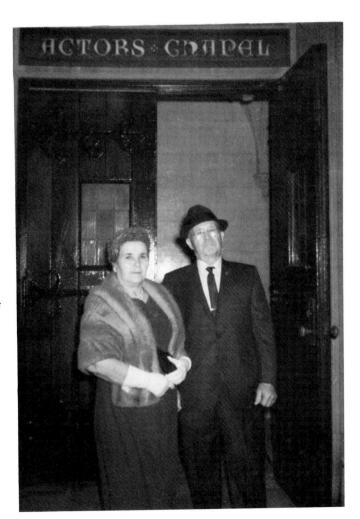

Mamma and Papa when we got married.

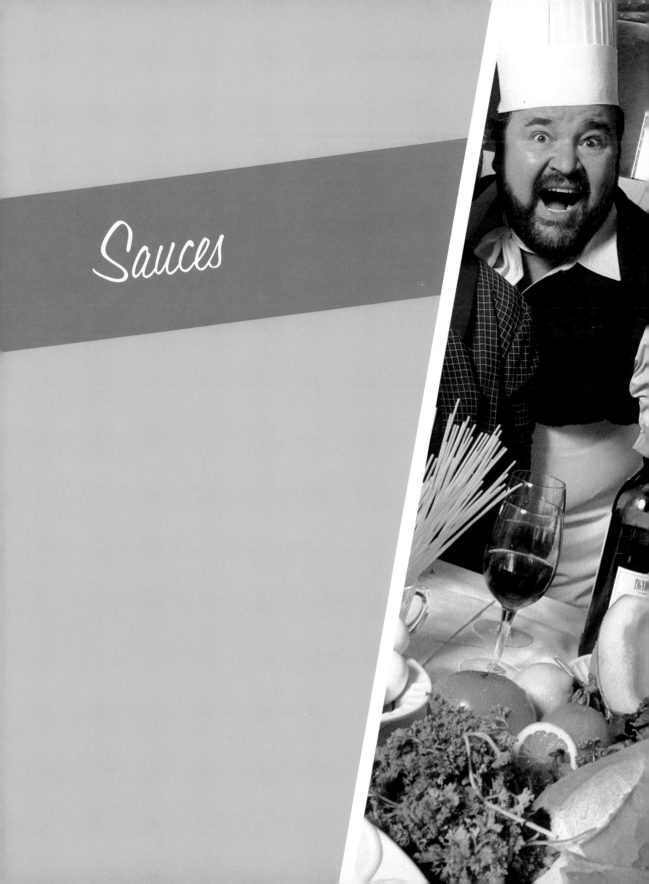

Sauces

MAMMA'S SUNDAY SAUCE

This is the sauce I grew up with, folks. It's got everything but the kitchen sink and the taste is oh, sooo good!

4	*garlic cloves*
1	*small onion, peeled, chopped*
4	*tablespoons olive oil*
10	*Italian sausages*
20	*meatballs (see Dom's Mom's Meatballs, page 164)*
6	*pork spareribs*
1	*Braciole (large piece of beef, chuck or round) placed between 2 pieces of wax paper and pounded thin, sprinkled with bread crumbs, grated cheese, basil, rolled and secured with toothpicks*

1	*pound boneless pork (no fat), in 1 piece*
6–8	*28-oz. cans crushed tomatoes*
1	*12-oz. can tomato paste*
1	*tablespoon sugar*
10	*large fresh basil leaves, coarsely chopped*
1	*teaspoon oregano*
	grated cheese

In a huge pot (I prefer stainless steel or enamel—not aluminum), gently fry garlic and onion in the oil until golden brown. Brown sausages in the same pan and set aside. Have browned meatballs ready. Brown the Braciole, set aside. Brown ribs and pork and set aside. Pour off the fat and add tomatoes and tomato paste. Gently heat to boiling, stirring often.

To the hot sauce add the meats, sugar, 5 basil leaves, and oregano.

Stir gently, let simmer for 2 hours, stirring occasionally. Skim off as much fat as you can and discard. Cut meats into serving portions. (If you are refrigerating this sauce before use, even better. All the fat can very easily be removed from the top when cold.) It's perfect on:

Homemade pasta	Fusilli	Angel hair	Manicotti
Lasagne	Rigatoni	Fettuccine	Wood Chips
Ravioli	Ziti	Linguine	

Sprinkle with additional chopped basil and grated cheese.

SERVES EVERYBODY WHO WALKS IN THE DOOR!

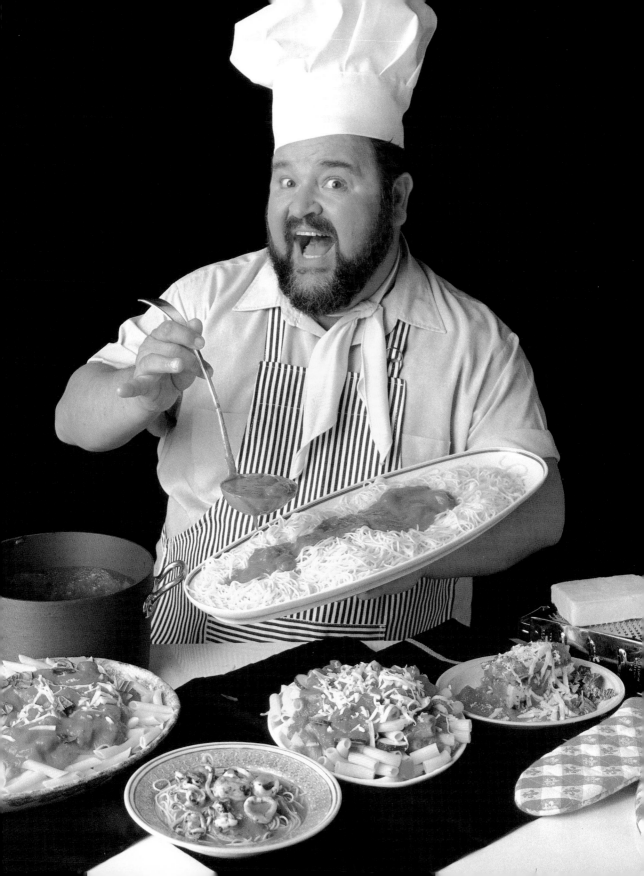

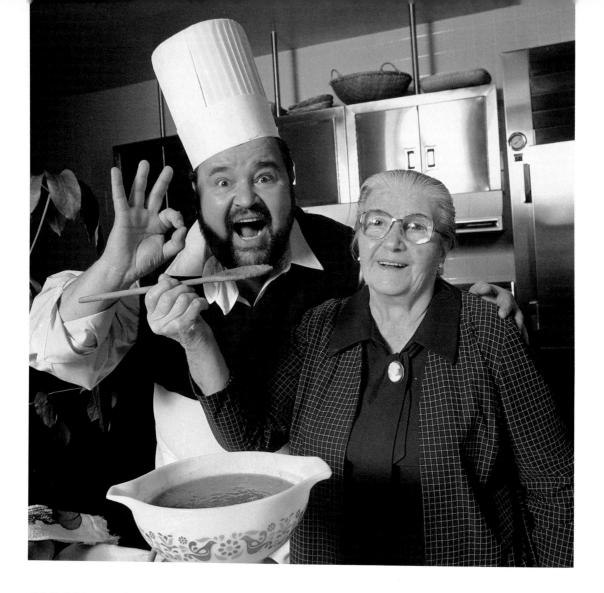

MAMMA'S MARINARA SAUCE

Mariner means sailor, but it's the sailors' wives who would wait for
their husbands to return home that gave this sauce its name. It's fresh
and delicious, but the best part is that it can easily be made while your
pasta water is boiling. The traditional marinara sauce calls for oil,
garlic, slices of peeled fresh tomatoes, and fresh basil, cooked for
about 20 minutes. It's fabulous sprinkled with grated cheese.
Mamma's Marinara Sauce takes a little longer to cook. I guess Papa's
ship was farther out. And Mamma's nontraditional addition of sun-
dried tomatoes really enhances the taste.

 4 *tablespoons olive oil*
 5 *garlic cloves, minced*
 2 *28-oz. cans ready-cut peeled tomatoes or 5 pounds fresh tomatoes,*
    peeled and sliced
 1 *6-oz. can tomato paste*
 4 *tablespoons sun-dried tomatoes, chopped (optional)*
10 *fresh basil leaves*
    pepper
    grated cheese

In a deep 10-inch frying pan, heat the olive oil and gently sauté the garlic. Add tomatoes, tomato paste and sun-dried tomatoes, if you are using these.

Put on medium heat for 20 to 30 minutes, stirring occasionally. Tear basil leaves into small pieces and sprinkle on top after adding to pasta. Add pepper and grated cheese to taste.

This sauce is fabulous with fish, scallops, shrimp, or broiled chicken, etc.

Alternative: Add 1 medium onion, finely chopped, and sauté the onion with the garlic until limp.

Each step makes a different sauce that is delicious, fresh and unique!

Note: If fresh tomatoes are used, put them in a pot of boiling water for about 10 seconds until the skin can be easily peeled off. Discard skin. Cut tomatoes into pieces and add to frying-pan mixture. Add tomato paste and sun-dried tomatoes.

MAKES ABOUT 2 QUARTS OF SAUCE.

MAMMA'S (AND MICHAEL'S) MEAT SAUCE

Once when my mother came to visit us, she taught my son Michael (who was nine years old at the time) to make this sauce. Michael (who is seventeen now) has been making it ever since. He takes requests for "Michael's Meat Sauce" without batting an eye.

4 *tablespoons olive oil*
1 *onion, chopped*
1 *carrot, chopped fine*
3 *cloves garlic, minced*
2 *28-oz. cans ready-cut, peeled tomatoes*
1 *6-oz. can tomato paste*
1 *teaspoon black pepper*
1 *teaspoon sugar*
1 *pound lean ground beef*
1 *teaspoon thyme*
10 *fresh mushrooms, diced*

In a saucepan, heat oil and lightly brown onion, carrot, and garlic. Stir in tomatoes, tomato paste, pepper, and sugar. Simmer gently for about 30 minutes.

While sauce is simmering, brown ground beef in skillet over medium-high heat, drain off fat. Add meat and thyme to tomato mixture. Cover and simmer ½ hour, stirring occasionally. Add mushrooms and cook another 10 minutes.

Great with 1 pound of pasta, cooked al dente.

SERVES 4–6.

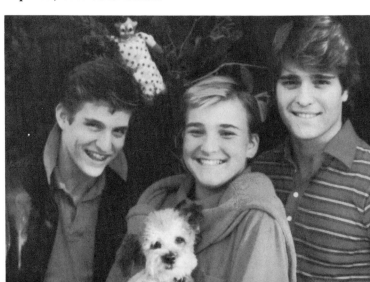

Michael, Midnight, David, and Peter, 1985.

MAMMA'S SPAGHETTI SAUCE
WITH ITALIAN SAUSAGE

You can serve this with or without pasta. But whatever your
pleasure, just don't come to dinner without a loaf of bread under each
arm.

1 ½	*pounds Italian sausage, hot or sweet*
¼	*cup hot water*
10–12	*fresh mushrooms, sliced*
1	*carrot, cut in half (this adds sweetness)*
1	*onion, minced*
2	*tablespoons olive oil*
2	*28-oz. cans ready-cut, peeled tomatoes*
1	*6-oz. can tomato paste*
1	*cup dry red wine*
3	*tablespoons fresh parsley, chopped*
1	*teaspoon basil*
½	*teaspoon oregano*
	freshly ground black pepper to taste

Place sausage in a skillet. Add hot water, cover and cook for 10
minutes. Remove sausages and separate the links.

Discard sausage drippings. In a large Dutch oven sauté mushrooms,
carrot, and onion just until al dente.

Add tomatoes, tomato paste, wine, parsley, basil, oregano and
pepper. Cover and simmer 1 hour or until thickened, stirring
occasionally.

Great with 1 to 1½ pounds of ziti, rigatoni, ravioli, or angel hair.

SERVES 6–8.

DOM'S AGLIO E OLIO
(Garlic and Oil)

My mother is known for having the fastest pan in Brooklyn. You can
make her Aglio e Olio with three simple ingredients in minutes: oil,
garlic, pasta. The dish tastes great cooked in this traditional way. But
over the years I have experimented, and this recipe has evolved . . .
and so far, I ain't heard no complaints.

½ cup olive oil
3   garlic cloves, minced
½ cup pignoli (pine nuts), coarsely chopped (optional)
½ cup walnuts or pecans, coarsely chopped (optional)
1   pound pasta (spaghettini, vermicelli, or other thin pasta)
2   tablespoons fresh parsley, chopped
4   basil leaves, coarsely torn
    freshly ground pepper
    grated cheese to taste

Heat oil in a small saucepan over low heat and very gently sauté garlic
and nuts until garlic is golden brown.
　　Cook pasta al dente. Pour into large, preheated serving bowl. Toss
quickly with garlic, nuts, and oil. Add parsley, basil, pepper and
grated cheese. Serve immediately.

SERVES 4–6.

PUTTANESCA SAUCE
(Harlot Sauce)

I did a show called "The Entertainers" with Caterina Valente, who made this "harlot" sauce for me and all the gypsies. ("Gypsies" is a theatrical term referring to all those hardworking singers and dancers in the show.) Caterina made an enormous pot of the sauce, and I can remember there wasn't a drop left, which is a great testimony to its flavor and her cooking . . . even though everyone in the theater knows that gypsies will eat anything, God love them. Bon appetite!

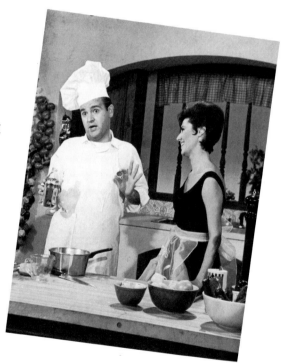

2 *garlic cloves, minced*
2 *tablespoons olive oil*
2 *28-oz. cans Italian plum tomatoes, whole*
1 *16-oz. can pitted whole black olives, drained*
4 *tablespoons capers, drained*
6 *fresh basil leaves, chopped*
  pinch of red pepper flakes

Sauté garlic in the oil until soft and golden brown. Add the tomatoes, simmer for 10 minutes. Add olives, capers, basil and red pepper. Simmer in uncovered pot for 20 minutes, stirring it gently until sauce has thickened. Great on 1 pound vermicelli cooked al dente.

Serve with cheese and wine. Excellent for gypsies, harlots, starlets, and friends.

SERVES 4–5.

CHICKEN (EASY DOES IT) SAUCE

Here's another fine dish my conductor's wife, Geri Sicari, got me into. The recipe's so easy you can phone it in. Geri leaves the chicken skin on, I take it off. But I promise you something that is juicy, tasty, tender and succulent—somebody kiss me!

2 chickens, cut up and skin removed
2 large onions, sliced thinly into rings
3 28-oz. cans crushed tomatoes
  fresh basil
  pepper
2 pounds spaghetti
1 cup grated Parmesan cheese

Place the chicken pieces in a baking pan or casserole dish. Arrange onion rings on top of chicken. Cover chicken with the crushed tomatoes. Sprinkle with basil and pepper.

Cook at 375 degrees for 1 hour and 20 minutes. Serve over spaghetti with Parmesan cheese sprinkled on top.

The onions and the chicken do something to the sauce that is unique and special. It's a real crowd pleaser—honest!

SERVES 8–10.

MAMMA'S EGGPLANT SAUCE

Not all Italians know about this sauce because the Neapolitans want to keep this secret for themselves. When you try it, you'll understand why!

1   *medium eggplant, peeled and cut into 1-inch cubes*
2   *tablespoons flour*
2   *garlic cloves, minced*
6   *tablespoons olive oil*
1   *onion, chopped*
2   *28-oz. cans crushed tomatoes*
1   *6-oz. can tomato paste*
6   *leaves fresh basil, chopped*
    black pepper
½   *teaspoon sugar*
    grated cheese

Sprinkle eggplant cubes with flour and toss to coat well; set aside.

In a large saucepan, heat oil and add eggplant. Brown lightly, stirring frequently. Remove eggplant to absorbent paper to drain.

Place garlic and onion in the saucepan, adding a little more oil if necessary, and cook until lightly browned. Stir in tomatoes, tomato paste, basil, pepper, and sugar. Simmer gently, uncovered, for 15 minutes, stirring occasionally. Add eggplant and heat gently, covered, 15 to 20 minutes longer, or until eggplant is fork-tender.

Serve over 1 pound spaghetti (cooked al dente), with Parmesan cheese.

Optional: Zucchini and carrots cut into 1-inch pieces added at the same time as eggplant. Good enough to serve as a side dish.

SERVES 4–6.

RED CLAM SAUCE FOR DINO

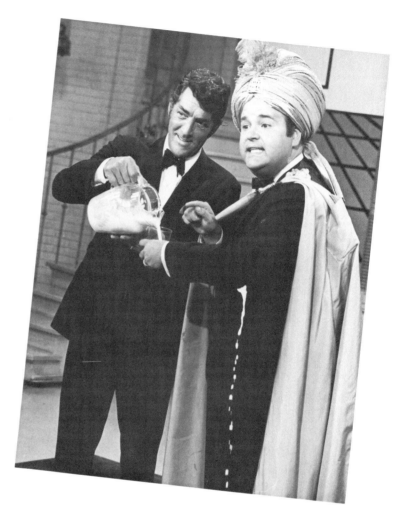

Dean Martin is a fabulous performer. I love the way he sings, he is hysterically funny, and what amazes me is how relaxed he is. He's been a good friend to me and a joy to work with for a lot of years.

I've often seen him work in Las Vegas, and the audience always has the feeling that he's just invited them into his living room for a casual evening—until the marvelous show's over and they realize a consummate professional was "easy" at work. The audience invariably gives him a standing ovation, which makes him happy as a clam.

Everybody wants to know if Dean drinks anymore. Well, I'll tell you . . . he doesn't drink any *less!* But one thing, for sure, that Dean can't get enough of is linguine with Red Clam Sauce!

4   tablespoons olive oil
4   garlic cloves, minced
1/2   teaspoon oregano
4   leaves of fresh basil, chopped
1   teaspoon chopped fresh parsley
1/4   teaspoon thyme
       pepper to taste
2   28-oz. cans ready-cut, peeled tomatoes
1   8-oz. bottle clam juice
1/2   cup dry white wine
5–6 6-oz. cans chopped clams
1 1/2 pounds pasta
       grated cheese

In a saucepan, gently heat the oil and sauté the garlic until golden brown. Add the oregano, basil, parsley, thyme, pepper, tomatoes, clam juice, and white wine. Bring to a boil and then reduce heat and simmer gently, uncovered, for 1 hour.

Ten minutes before serving, add the clams and heat gently until ready. In the meantime, cook the pasta al dente. I find it best to take half of the sauce (the most liquid part) and mix with the hot pasta, tossing gently, and then making individual servings. Now, ladle generous heapings of the dense, clam-filled sauce on the individual servings. Perfect! Oh, and of course, grated cheese is okay!

SERVES 6–8.

Note: If you can find some, and feel like splurging, substitute fresh clams for the canned, cooking them in the sauce just until they open. Allow 6–10 clams per person.

WHITE CLAM SAUCE À LA PEGGY

My very special friend, Peggy Mondo, was in the movie *Fatso* with me. She and her mother fed the entire cast and crew with the best clam sauce I've ever tasted. She taught me everything I know about clams, and a lot more about people. My life is better because of her, and so is my white clam sauce.

½   *cup olive oil*
10 *garlic cloves, minced*
2   *8-oz. bottles of clam juice*
    juice of 1 lemon
1   *cup dry white wine*
1   *tablespoon oregano*
4   *tablespoons fresh parsley, minced*
4   *leaves fresh basil, coarsely chopped*
6   *6-oz. cans chopped clams, or 1 46-oz. can*
1½ *pounds linguine or angel hair*

Heat the garlic very gently in the oil to a golden brown. Add the clam juice, the lemon juice, the wine, oregano, and parsley and heat thoroughly about 20 minutes; keep hot.

In the meantime, cook pasta al dente. A moment before you drain your pasta, add the basil and the clams to the hot clam juice mixture (the clams will stay nice and tender). Drain the pasta and put it in a hot serving bowl, along with half the liquid, then make individual servings. Now ladle generous heapings of the clam-filled sauce on the individual servings. It's kinda so they won't be searching for the clams. They'll be right there. Orgasmic!

In Naples, my waiter forbid us to use grated cheese because it might mar the subtle taste of the clams. I do like this better without the cheese. But as far as I'm concerned, do what you like!

Clam lovers of the world, unite!

SERVES 6–8.

Note: Fresh clams? See *note* in Red Clam Sauce, page 129.

MOM'S MUSSELS MARINARA WITH MOSTACCIOLI

This is special, and you can use any pasta that tickles your palate. I just like mostaccioli, and it starts with an "M." Mostaccioli are just like ziti. I love to use a mussel shell to scoop up this scrumptious sauce.

1   *quart mussels in their shells*
3   *tablespoons olive oil*
1   *small onion, chopped*
4   *garlic cloves, minced*
2   *28-oz. cans ready-cut, peeled tomatoes*
½   *teaspoon oregano*
    dash of red pepper
    dash of black pepper
1   *16-oz. can black olives, drained and pitted*
½   *cup chopped parsley*
½   *cup dry white wine*
1   *pound mostaccioli*
1   *cup fresh basil leaves, coarsely torn*

Scrub mussels with a stiff brush under running water until clean, and scrape off their "beards."

Heat oil in a Dutch oven over medium heat. Add onion and garlic and cook until golden brown. Add tomatoes, oregano, red pepper, black pepper, olives, parsley, and wine. Cook on medium heat, uncovered, for about 15 minutes, stirring occasionally. Then add mussels and stir to coat with sauce. Cover and simmer just until mussels have opened (6–8 minutes). Discard any that don't open.

Cook mostaccioli al dente, and place in large serving bowl. Pour mussels and sauce over pasta, and mix gently so all pasta is coated with sauce. Sprinkle with fresh basil leaves.

Your mouth will thank you—trust me!

SERVES 4–6.

MAMMA'S SEAFOOD SAUCE

I suggest you wear a giant plastic bib around your mouth, face and ears, because when you taste this you are going to want to dive in!

4 *tablespoons olive oil*
2 *onions, minced*
4 *cloves garlic, minced*
1 *cup dry white wine*
4 *28-oz. cans ready-cut, peeled tomatoes*
4 *teaspoons fresh basil*
1 *tablespoon oregano*
4 *teaspoons fresh parsley, chopped*
3 *pounds small fresh clams, well scrubbed, or 4 cans chopped clams*
2 *pounds scallops, quartered*
2 *pounds shrimp, peeled and deveined*
  black pepper

Heat the oil and sauté onions and garlic over medium-high heat until golden brown. Pour in wine and cook about 2 minutes.

Add tomatoes, basil, oregano, and parsley, and continue to cook over medium-high heat for another 5 minutes, then reduce heat to simmer. Cook for 30–40 minutes, until sauce is slightly thickened.

Add fresh clams, cover and cook until shells open, about 5 minutes. (If using canned clams, add at same time as shrimps and scallops.)

Add scallops and shrimps. Cover and cook until barely firm, about 3 minutes. Add pepper to taste. Remove from heat and serve immediately over pasta in large individual serving bowls.

Don't forget very large napkins . . . this is lip-smackin' good!

SERVES 12–?

CALAMARI AND SHELLFISH SAUCE

Our family goes mad for this recipe! It makes any evening seem like Christmas Eve, even when you make it in July.

18	*fresh cherrystone clams, scrubbed*
3	*pounds mussels, scrubbed and beards removed*
1	*cup red wine*
1	*onion, chopped*
8–10	*garlic cloves, minced*
½	*cup olive oil*
4	*28-oz. cans ready-cut, peeled tomatoes*
1	*teaspoon oregano*
3	*teaspoons fresh basil*
3–4	*tablespoons parsley*
	pepper to taste
2	*pounds calamari (squid), cleaned and sliced (see page 182)*
1	*pound large shrimp, cleaned and deveined*
	red pepper flakes (optional)
2	*pounds linguine*

Some of the DeLuise clan on Mamma's eighty-eighth birthday, 1987.

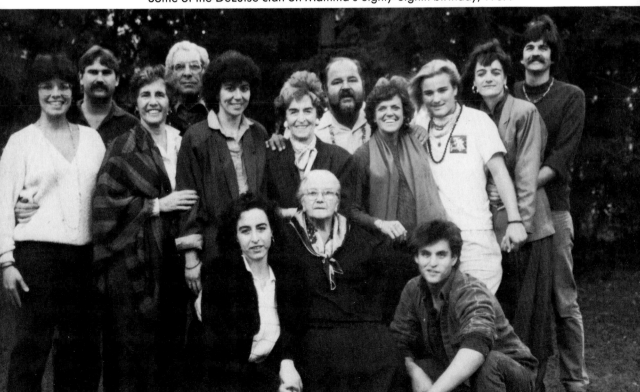

In a large pot, steam clams and mussels in ½ cup red wine until they open. Discard any that don't open. Set aside and keep warm.

In a large Dutch oven, sauté the onion and garlic in the olive oil. Add tomatoes, oregano, basil, parsley, remaining ½ cup red wine, salt and pepper, and simmer about 20 minutes. Add the calamari, shrimp, mussels, and clams (with broth) and cook 5 minutes more, or until shrimp are done. Serve over linguine. Add crushed red pepper, if desired.

This is quick and easy and delicious once ingredients are assembled.

SERVES 8–10.

SCANDALOUS SCALLOP SAUCE

Ernie Chambers is a producer and a good friend. His wife, Veronica, is vivacious and a really fine cook. The night she made this dish for us, she said it is great on pasta, but decided to serve it without. Silly woman, doesn't she know I like *everything* on pasta? She was pleased when I asked her for this recipe and I carefully wrote down everything she said.

1   tablespoon olive oil
4   garlic cloves, minced
2   shallots
4   leaves fresh basil, chopped
2   teaspoons fresh parsley, chopped
1   teaspoon fresh thyme
2   quarts of fresh tomatoes, skinned and chopped
      (or 2 28-oz. cans of plum tomatoes)
½ cup white wine
1   pound mushrooms, quartered
4   tablespoons olive oil
1   teaspoon butter
2   pounds small scallops
1   tablespoon lemon juice
      pepper
1   pound linguine, cooked

In a large pot, heat oil and briefly sauté the garlic and shallots. Add the basil, parsley, thyme, tomatoes and wine. Bring to a boil and simmer for 20 minutes. Then add mushrooms.

In a frying pan, gently sauté the scallops in a little olive oil and butter. Add the lemon juice and pepper. (Cooks in minutes—don't overcook!)

Combine the sauce and scallops and serve immediately over hot pasta, or serve on rice, or even by itself in small individual casserole dishes. You can't go wrong.

SERVES 8.

Note: I made one change in this recipe. Veronica puts her garlic in at the end of the recipe. I put mine in at the beginning. I just feel it works better, I'm not apologizing.

Rice and

Other Grains

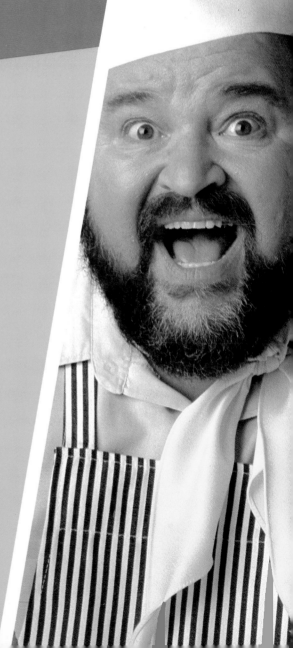

NOT WITH *MY* FORK!

When I was a kid I had chores, like cutting the bread, grating the cheese, and setting the table—and when I set the table I would always make sure that I would get my favorite fork. This fork had a plastic handle which fit just right in my hand, and real sharp prongs, so when my mother made risotto it would pick up every single kernel. It was perfect. I *loved* that fork!

As you can imagine, our house always smelled as if the cooking had been going on for days and days. And it had! During the hot summer months Mamma would open the windows for air so that even a "bum" could get a free meal by simply following his nose. You understand, there is no one more generous than an Italian after supper, and Mamma was *always* kind. I remember once a bum came to the door and asked my mom for a meal. Much to my chagrin, she gave him *my favorite fork* to eat with. I didn't say anything but I knew that I would never use that fork again. It was ruined! I stood there horrified! How could she do this to me? There could be no way to erase the memory of this hobo eating with my favorite fork.

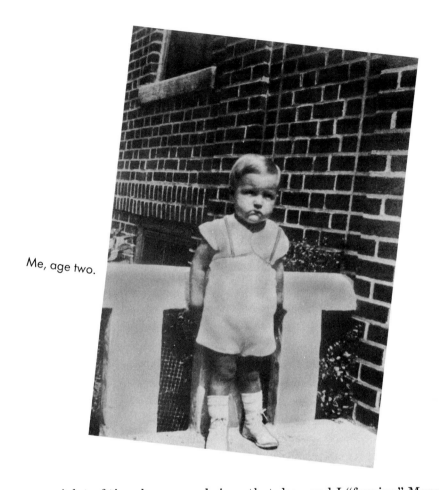

Me, age two.

A lot of time has passed since that day, and I "forgive" Mamma for
what she did because her heart was in the right place. I'm an adult
and I use any old fork to eat with now. Know what I mean? I guess it
was time I gave up on my fork. Sometimes though, I wonder
whatever happened to "forkie." Where is he now? What's he doing?
Scrambling eggs? Digging into some Caesar salad? Is he off
somewhere doing crazy things to a crepe Suzette? Eh, we had a lot of
good times together. C'est la vie! All I can say is that it's a good thing
my mamma's risotto was so delicious. I could eat that with *any* old
fork!

RISOTTO

There are even some Italians who don't know about the joys of risotto. But it's very traditional Italian fare; and it's high in carbohydrates and low in fat. The only trick is making enough.

4–5 cups chicken broth
2   tablespoons olive oil
3   tablespoons butter
1   small onion, finely chopped
1½ cups Italian short-grained pearl rice (or rice of your choice)
¼   cup freshly grated cheese

Bring the chicken broth to simmering. Heat the olive oil and 2 tablespoons of the butter over medium-high heat in a heavy, deep frying pan. Sauté the onion until soft and lightly golden. Stir in the rice and sauté about 2 minutes until well coated with oil and butter. Add ½ cup of the simmering broth. Keep liquid simmering and stir continually, scraping the bottom and sides of the pan until the liquid has evaporated.

Add more hot broth, ½ cup at a time, whenever the rice becomes dry, and stir continually. You may not need all the broth before the rice is done . . . or you may need a little more, so in that case just add a little water. Cook the rice until it's tender, but a little firm to the bite. The rice should be creamy but not soupy. Total simmering time should run about 30 to 35 minutes.

A couple of minutes before you think the rice is done, stir in the cheese and remaining tablespoon of butter. Serve immediately with grated cheese sprinkled on top of each serving.

SERVES 4.

RISOTTO PRIMAVERA

Just like pasta, this risotto stands alone as a first course.

4   *cups chicken broth*
3   *tablespoons olive oil*
3   *tablespoons butter*
2   *onions, chopped*
2   *celery stalks, chopped*
2   *carrots, chopped*
1   *cup fresh parsley, chopped*
6–8 *fresh basil leaves, chopped*
2   *cups Italian short-grained pearl rice (or rice of your choice)*
8–10 *plum tomatoes, diced*
2   *small zucchini, sliced thin*
1   *cup peas*
¼   *cup freshly grated Parmesan cheese*

Bring the chicken broth to simmering. Heat the olive oil and the butter over medium-high heat in a heavy, deep frying pan. Sauté the onions until soft and lightly golden. Stir in the celery, carrots, parsley, basil, and rice, and sauté about 2 minutes until well coated with oil and butter. Add ½ cup of the simmering broth. Keep liquid simmering and stir continually, scraping the bottom and sides of the pan, until the liquid has been absorbed.

Add the tomatoes, zucchini, peas, and another ½ cup of the hot broth, and stir continually. Each time the rice becomes dry, add another ½ cup of broth. You may not need all the liquid before the rice is done . . . or you may need a little more, so in that case just add water. Cook the rice until it's tender, but a little firm to the bite. Total simmering time should run about 30 to 35 minutes.

Serve with a bowl of grated Parmesan cheese in case someone wants to sprinkle some over their dish.

SERVES 6.

BROWN RICE LOUISE

My friend and writing partner, Maurice Richlin, who wrote *Pillow Talk*, was on the Brown Rice Diet, and one day after an intense writing session, his wife, Louise, walked in with this. After licking the bowl clean, I convinced her to give me the recipe, which I'll now share with you. It's nutritious, tasty and *wonderful!* (Oh, by the way, my son Michael loves this for breakfast.)

1 cup brown rice
2 cups water or chicken stock
1 pat butter

1 large onion, chopped
1 large green apple, chopped

Cook rice in water or chicken stock and set aside. In a nonstick pan, sauté onion in butter until transparent. Add chopped green apple. Brown together for five minutes. Add the cooked rice and heat, tossing gently.

SERVES 4–6.

GRAINS, BREAKFAST, LUNCH, DINNER

I have a friend, Bill Metzger, who is very tall and very thin. He runs eight miles every day and has these mixed grains for breakfast. I expressed an interest in them, and the next day he arrived on my doorstep with a huge jarful. They have been a sensational addition to my kitchen. That jar is constantly being replenished. Now, I don't run eight miles, but I do use the grains. Eh! You can't have everything. These grains are very nutritious and everyone who tastes them gets turned on.

In my kitchen, stored in a cool, dry place, there is a huge jar that contains:

1 pound brown rice
1 pound wheat
1 pound barley

½ pound bulgur wheat
½ pound millet
(all mixed)

Cook 1 cup of mixed grains to 2 cups of liquid (water or broth). This amount will serve 4. Cook more, proportionately, as needed. When simmered over a low flame, and all the liquid is absorbed, you have a delicious, nutty, crunchy taste that is absolutely scrumptious just as is. It's also good in the morning with milk and sugar. You can even add diced apples, raisins and cinnamon.

When you cook the grains in chicken broth, it's an excellent accompaniment to meat, fish, chicken, with steamed vegetables, or added to soups.

Try it! It's delicious, cheap, convenient, and healthy!

BASIC POLENTA

Polenta is very popular in Italy, and leftovers, which have a very firm consistency, can be fried like grits. Very few people know this, but polenta can be used to repair broken stucco and any cracks in your home! The nice part is, when you're hungry, all you've got to do is lick the walls. Seriously, though, the real trick here is to keep stirring it slowly . . . and keep believing.

6   *cups water*
2   *cups polenta, or coarse-grained cornmeal*

Bring water to a boil in a heavy saucepan. Reduce heat so water is just simmering and gradually add the polenta in a steady stream. Stir constantly.

Continue to stir until polenta is thickened. Polenta should come away from the sides of the pan and be able to support a spoon. Pour thickened polenta onto a wooden board and let stand for a few minutes before turning out onto a serving platter.

Polenta can be served in a variety of ways: as a bed for chicken, sausages, or rabbit stew. As a first course, it can be topped with grated cheese. Polenta is delicious served with marinara sauce too . . . just make indentations and fill the wells with your favorite spaghetti sauce. Have fun serving your polenta by cutting it the "old-fashioned" way: hold a string tautly and slice right through.

SERVES 5–6.

Poultry and Rabbit

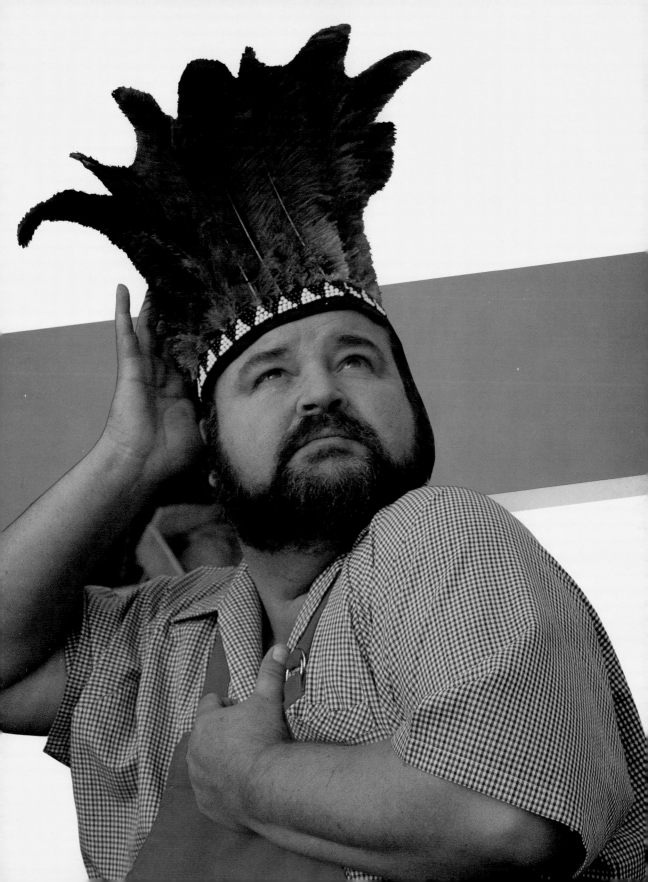

STAY PREGNANT

I remember sitting at the dinner table as a child, with my feet not touching the floor, listening to stories my family and relatives would tell over their after-dinner espresso. The stories would go on for hours. Sometimes they were sad, and people would cry, but more often than not the stories were very funny, leaving my mom weak from laughter. One story I loved, no matter how many times I heard it: The story was about my mother trying to "stay pregnant."

One of the things that mothers do is they get pregnant and give birth to children. Being Catholic and Italian and having no television, my mother did this a lot. My brother Nick was born in 1921, and my sister Anne in 1926. After that, my mother had some miscarriages and had difficulty staying pregnant. So when my mother suspected she was pregnant with me, she went to see Doctor Tomasuola, who informed her that she was in a very delicate condition, and if she wanted this baby to go to full term, she shouldn't climb stairs, she should have complete bed rest, and above all, she should *have no excitement*. So that evening my father, in an effort to follow the doctor's orders, did his best to take care of my brother Nick and my sister Anne, and told my mother to go to bed, relax completely, and that he would make dinner.

My mother had been resting for fifteen minutes when my father came home with two live chickens. (At that time, you went to the chicken market, bought a live chicken, took it home, killed it, dressed it, and cooked it.) While my mother was in bed as per doctor's orders, my father took these two chickens into the bathroom. I guess he didn't close the door very well, because after he slit both their throats, they somehow escaped. So in this tiny Brooklyn apartment, there were two chickens running around, literally like chickens with their heads cut off . . . leaving a trail of blood everywhere: on the drapes, couches, rugs, and all through the kitchen! My father tried desperately to catch them, yelling all the while to my mother, "Yousa be calms, no movesa, jasta relaxa and stays in bed". . . he would take care of everything! Meanwhile he was covered with blood, the chickens were flapping their wings and the apartment was getting redecorated in red. Needless to say, in spite of Papa's "assistance," Mamma got up, and they cleaned the apartment together. That was the end of doctor's orders. She spent the rest of the day cleaning up, cooking, washing, and generally tidying up the place so that no one would know that two chickens had their swan song there. The whole experience must have done Mamma good, because a few months later, I was born bright and healthy and weighed in at eight pounds eight ounces.

When retelling this story, even my father laughed, in spite of himself—but it's my mamma who always laughed the most!

Now, for you hearty souls, here are my favorite chicken recipes.

MAMMA'S CHICKEN

My mother serves this from the stove to the table piping hot. It really has an extra zesty flavor if you serve it with a wedge of lemon that you squeeze on the chicken just before eating. Just thinking about it makes my mouth water!

2 chickens, cut up in serving pieces
1 cup lemon juice
2 cups seasoned bread crumbs mixed with
2 tablespoons grated cheese
1 onion, sliced
  olive oil

Dip chicken in lemon juice, and then roll in seasoned bread-crumb-and-cheese mixture. In a baking dish, place onion in and around chicken. Sprinkle with olive oil and bake in preheated 350-degree oven for 1 hour, uncovered.
  Serve immediately.

SERVES 6–8.

Variation: My mother does the same thing with potatoes. You take 4 potatoes, peeled and cut in sixths lengthwise. Rub a little olive oil on each piece, dip in seasoned bread crumbs mixed with cheese and place between chicken pieces. You can even cook the potatoes in a baking dish of their own at 350 degrees for 1 hour. They are a perfect accompaniment to roast beef, veal, or pork. Kids love them because they're like a giant french fry.

CHICKEN DOMINICK

This is special and might even be called "Mock Veal." It is delicious served with wild rice, asparagus, a mixed green salad with olive oil and lemon juice, and hot French bread. *Shazam!*

4 chicken breasts, split and boned
  flour
1 garlic clove
  butter
1 large green pepper, sliced
1 large red pepper, sliced
8 mushrooms, sliced
5 tablespoons sauterne

Place chicken breasts between 2 pieces of wax paper, pound them so they look like cutlets, and dredge in flour. Sauté garlic in butter, remove when brown. Add chicken breasts and sauté 1 minute on each side. Add green and red peppers, mushrooms, and wine. Shake the pan. Cover and simmer for 15 minutes.

SERVES 4.

NANCY REAGAN'S BAJA CALIFORNIA CHICKEN

When we were compiling this cookbook, this was the first recipe my editor tried out, and he said, "Dom, I tried Nancy Reagan's chicken, and you know something . . . it was good!" The President and my editor have enjoyed this chicken, and now, so can you.

8	*chicken breasts, boned*
	salt and pepper
2	*cloves garlic, crushed*
4	*tablespoons olive oil*
4	*tablespoons tarragon vinegar*
⅔	*cup sherry*

Sprinkle chicken with salt and pepper. Add crushed garlic to oil and vinegar in a skillet. Sauté chicken pieces until golden brown, turning frequently, about 10 minutes.

Pour sherry over the chicken and place skillet in preheated 350-degree oven for 10 minutes.

SERVES 2 REPUBLICANS, 2 AMBASSADORS, 2 DIGNITARIES, AND MR. AND MRS. TIP O'NEILL—8.

LONI'S CHICKEN WITH WILD RICE

Loni Anderson is one of the prettiest women I've ever known. She is a very funny comedienne, and she's very good in the kitchen. She's been real nice to a certain friend of mine . . . but leave us not digress!

2	*cups wild rice, uncooked*
1	*green pepper, coarsely chopped*
1	*red pepper, coarsely chopped*
3	*ribs celery, coarsely chopped*
1	*onion, chopped*
2	*cups chicken broth*
6	*chicken-breast halves, skin removed*
	soy sauce

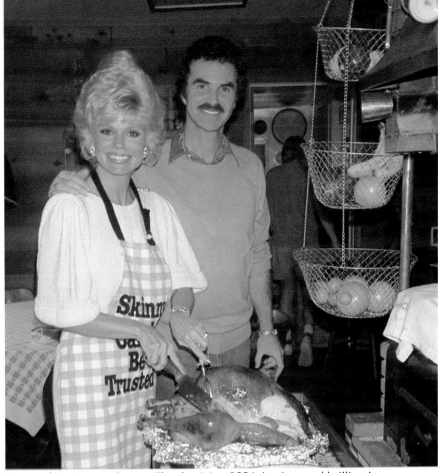

Burt and Loni at our house, Thanksgiving 1986. Loni carved brilliantly.

1   can cream of mushroom soup (trust me)
8–10   mushrooms, sliced
½   cup blanched almonds

Combine the rice with the peppers, celery, onion, and chicken broth in a 9-by-11-inch casserole. Cover and bake at 350 degrees for 40 minutes.

Brush chicken breasts with soy sauce; immerse in rice.

In a mixing bowl, combine cream of mushroom soup with mushrooms and almonds. Pour over chicken-and-rice mixture. Mix slightly and bake covered for another 40 minutes.

SERVES 6.

DOM'S GINGER CHICKEN

I like to serve this dish for company. Don't worry about the ginger taste being too strong and taking over. The sour cream puts the ginger in its place, and it's a marriage made in heaven.

1 stick of butter (¼ pound)
2 tablespoons freshly grated ginger
2 bunches scallions, chopped
1 cup chicken stock
4 whole boneless chicken breasts, cut into bite-sized pieces
2 cans water chestnuts, drained and sliced
1 pound fresh button mushrooms, quartered
   pepper to taste
3 cups sour cream
6 cups cooked brown or white rice
   chopped parsley for garnish

Heat butter in a wok or large skillet. Sauté the ginger and scallions until the scallions are slightly wilted. Add the chicken stock and heat to near boiling. Add the chicken, reduce the heat and stir gently. Simmer until the chicken is *just* cooked. Add the water chestnuts, mushrooms, and pepper, and simmer for 2 minutes, stirring gently. Add 2 cups of the sour cream and continue stirring until blended thoroughly. Keep on a very *looooow* flame. Serve over rice with a dollop of sour cream on top of each serving. Sprinkle with fresh parsley.

SERVES 8–10.

MARIA'S PAELLA

For twenty years, Maria Iniguez has been our housekeeper, and she is like a member of our family. She is loving, a lot of fun, and very Spanish. Maria's Paella is her pièce de résistance! It's very festive, great for parties and the sing-alongs we always have at our house once this splendid dish has been consumed.

4   tablespoons olive oil
4   garlic cloves, chopped
1   chicken, cut in medium-sized pieces
6–8 mushrooms cut in pieces
4   Italian sausages
1   large onion, chopped
1   green pepper, sliced
1   red pepper, sliced
2   cups rice
2   cups boiling water
2   cups chicken stock
1   teaspoon saffron
1   cup fresh peas
8   mussels, scrubbed, beards removed
1   dozen clams, scrubbed
1   pound shrimp, peeled and deveined
1   can pimentos
    fresh parsley

In a large, deep skillet (or a paella pan if you have one), heat olive oil and garlic. Brown chicken lightly on a medium flame. Add mushrooms, sausages, onion, and green and red peppers. Cook 10 minutes over low heat and add rice. Cook 5 more minutes.

Add boiling water, chicken stock and saffron. Mix well and cook, covered, for 20 minutes or until liquid is absorbed. Add peas, mussels, clams and shrimp. Cook until mussels and clams open and shrimp turn pink. Garnish with pimentos and parsley.

SERVES 6–8.

ITALIAN FRIED RABBIT AND/OR CHICKEN
Here's Something Good!

When I was twenty-three years old, I was in New York doing an Off-Broadway show called *Little Mary Sunshine* at the Orpheum Theater, with Eileen Brennan. Dora Barnes, an elderly lady who lived across the street from the theater, just loved show folk, and each week she would feed our hungry cast between matinee and evening performances. Her wonderful menus varied, but somehow they always included rabbit. Since I was in the show for over a year, I got to taste rabbit *lots* of different ways.

1 *3-pound rabbit or chicken, cut up*
1 *egg*
1 *cup buttermilk*
1 *cup flour*
½ *cup grated cheese*
2 *garlic cloves, crushed*
¼ *teaspoon crushed dried basil leaves*
¼ *teaspoon dried oregano leaves*
¼ *teaspoon celery seed*
¼ *teaspoon dried marjoram leaves*
    oil for deep frying
    lemon wedges

Wash rabbit or chicken and pat dry. Beat egg in a bowl. Stir in buttermilk until well blended. Mix flour with grated cheese, garlic, basil, oregano, celery seed, and marjoram. Dip each piece of meat in egg-buttermilk mixture, then dredge in flour mixture.

Deep-fry, a few pieces at a time, until golden brown and tender. Drain on paper towels.

Squeeze some lemon wedges on the cooked pieces just before eating.

SERVES 4–6.

RABBIT CACCIATORE

You'll enjoy this today, and tomorrow it's even better!

6   *tablespoons olive oil*
4   *garlic cloves, minced*
1   *large onion, chopped*
2   *carrots, sliced*
8–10 *mushrooms, sliced*
3   *large tomatoes, chopped*
1   *8-oz. can tomato sauce*
½   *cup dry red wine*
2   *tablespoons minced oregano*
1   *teaspoon sugar*
1   *cup water*
      pepper
1   *rabbit, cut up*
2   *tablespoons butter or margarine*

Heat 4 tablespoons olive oil in skillet. Sauté garlic, onion, and carrots. Add mushrooms and continue to sauté. Add tomatoes and sauté. Add tomato sauce, wine, oregano, sugar, and water. Heat through. Season to taste with pepper.

Brown rabbit on both sides in mixture of the butter and remaining olive oil. Add rabbit to sauce. Cover and simmer about 35 minutes or until rabbit is tender. Uncover and continue cooking until sauce is thickened.

Serve as is or on brown rice or pasta.

SERVES 4.

STEWED RABBIT STEW

If you had two cups of wine, you'd be stewed too!

1	rabbit, cut into serving pieces
½	cup flour
2	tablespoons unsalted butter
4	garlic cloves, minced
	pepper
1	medium onion, sliced
2	medium carrots, peeled and sliced
8–10	mushrooms, sliced
2	large potatoes, quartered
1	bay leaf
½	teaspoon sage
½	teaspoon oregano
½	teaspoon thyme
½	teaspoon savory
½	teaspoon marjoram
	few sprigs parsley
2	cups dry red wine
1	cup water
2	tablespoons brown sugar
	parsley for garnish

Dust rabbit pieces with flour. Melt butter in a heavy skillet over medium heat. Add rabbit pieces and brown on all sides—this will take about 10 minutes. Add garlic, and pepper to taste. Add onions, carrots, mushrooms, potatoes, bay leaf, sage, oregano, thyme, savory, marjoram, parsley, and 1 cup of red wine.

Cover and simmer until vegetables are tender-crisp. Add remaining cup wine, water, and brown sugar. Cover and simmer over low heat, stirring as necessary, 30 to 45 minutes, or until sauce is of desired thickness. Remove bay leaf and garnish with more parsley.

SERVES 4.

Note: Chickens are great stewed, too.

RABBIT CON POLENTA

This dish is extremely popular in Venice and Naples, and will be at your home too!

2   tablespoons butter
2   tablespoons olive oil
1   rabbit, cut into pieces
2   stalks celery, sliced
1   carrot, sliced
1   medium onion, cut into
      small pieces
6–8 mushrooms, sliced
2   garlic cloves, crushed
2   sprigs of fresh rosemary
      or ½ teaspoon dried
2   whole cloves
1   cup Chianti or other dry red wine
1   cup chicken broth
      pepper
      polenta (see Basic Polenta, page 143)

Heat butter and oil in large heavy skillet. Add rabbit, turning frequently, until brown on both sides. Add celery, carrot, onion, mushrooms, garlic, rosemary, cloves, wine, and broth. Season with pepper. Cover and simmer over low heat until rabbit is very tender and meat pulls easily from bone, about 1 hour.

Serve on polenta.

SERVES 4–6.

Note: Polenta is also very kind to chicken and veal.

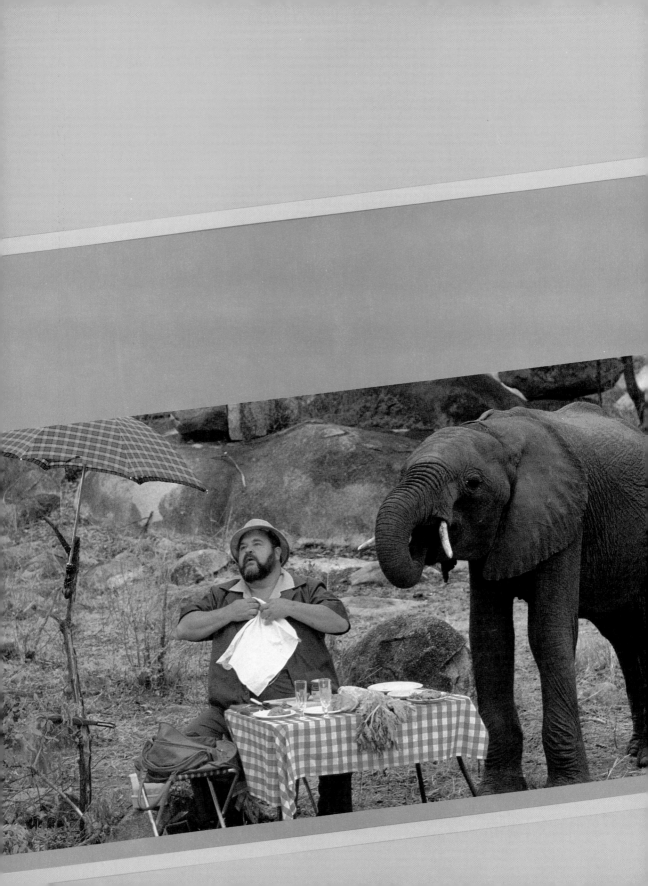

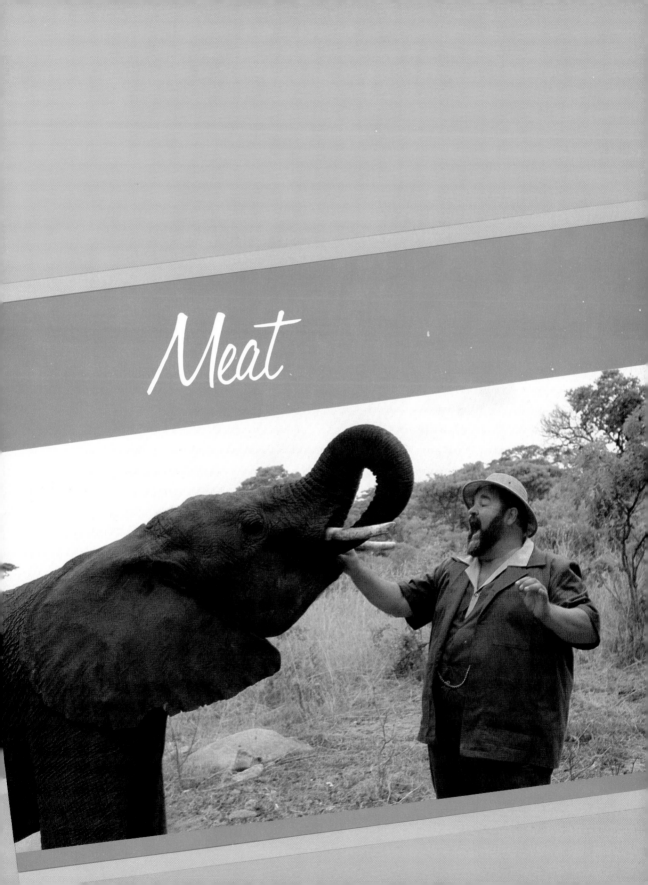

Meat

One of the things that is a jolt to your Catholic youth is that you have to confess your sins. Every Wednesday I would leave public school and go to catechism. The nuns would teach us about sins, and if you laughed, they'd rap your knuckles with a wooden ruler. In my teens, all nuns had their heads completely covered. I wasn't sure, but I assumed they were bald, and figured that was why they were so grouchy. When it was finally time for me to go to my first confession, I asked my cousin, Junior Degatano, "What do you tell the priest when you go in there . . . I mean, what are sins?" He was six months older than me so I figured he must really know. "Dom," he said, "you've got to tell the priest everything. If you ate meat on Friday . . . if you disobeyed your parents . . . if you did the puberty thing."

I said, "Oh, no, not the puberty thing. That's the best thing that happened to me since I got my teeth!" For those of you who don't know, there are different kinds of sins, venial and mortal. Venial is a small, insignificant kind of sin. Now a mortal sin, ha! . . . you enjoy more. Mortal sins are wonderful. They clear up your complexion. If you die with a mortal sin on your soul, you go straight to "Fun City"

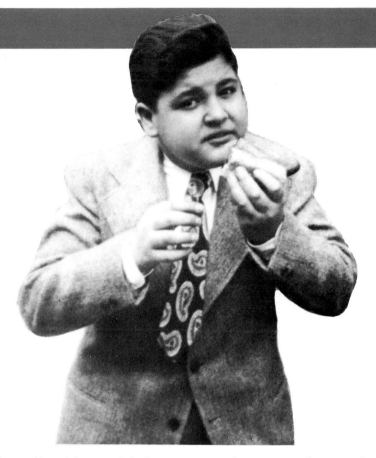

fast. If you die with a venial sin on your soul, you go to heaven, but you stop off in purgatory. Purgatory is like a Howard Johnson's along the way. It's all very complicated.

I remember one Friday a long time ago when I was a kid, I was having a hot dog and a Yoo-Hoo. It was a long time ago because the hot dog was 5 cents. I remember it was so delicious, the roll was so soft, the hot dog steaming, sauerkraut, mustard . . . ahh. I took my first bite. Just then my cousin came driving by on his bicycle, and when he saw what I was doing he skidded to a stop in horror. "Dom," he cried, "it's Friday." I didn't know what to do. I panicked . . . my little Italian heart was beating so fast. I didn't know if I should spit out the hot dog I had in my mouth and go absolutely clean, or swallow it and go for a venial. I mean, it really wasn't my fault, I didn't *realize* it was Friday. But the hot dog was so tasty, the roll was so hot, the sauerkraut . . . Anyway, I ate the whole thing and figured I'd go for a mortal.

Except for Fridays, our family enjoyed lots of sin-free meat, especially the veal and sausage dishes included here. Oh, life was simple when I was little. And it's not a sin to eat meat on Friday anymore. But then, it costs much more than 5 cents for a hot dog now, and that old neighborhood taste is gone. Besides, I have a sneaky feeling the mortal sin is what they put *in* the hot dog these days!

SAUSAGES WITH PEPPERS AND ONIONS

My mamma taught me the special trick to making this dish: When you're cooking, keep the skillet uncovered so the peppers and onions don't get steamed. Also—if you turn off the flame at just the right moment like Mamma does (that's the secret!) it'll make all the difference in the world. This dish is so special. Serve it with some hot Italian bread and a bottle of Chianti . . . some good friends and soft music . . . It will bring tears to your eyes!

Veal sausages can be used instead of pork sausages for an extra-special treat.

1½   pounds Italian sausages (sweet and/or hot, according to taste)
2   tablespoons olive oil
4   garlic cloves, minced
3   large onions, slivered
3   each, sweet red peppers and green peppers, seeded and cut into
*   strips*
½   teaspoon oregano

Pierce each sausage in several places with a fork and place in a heavy frying pan in 1 tablespoon of olive oil over medium-low heat. Turning occasionally, cook until well browned.

While sausages are cooking, add 1 tablespoon olive oil and sauté the garlic and the onion. Mix in the peppers and oregano. Cook until the onions are lightly brown and the peppers are tender. Place the sausages, peppers, and onions on a warm platter to serve.

SERVES 4–6.

MAMMA'S HOMEMADE SAUSAGE

There is a joke about a man who took his mother fishing. After a while she caught a fish, reeled it in, looked at it, and immediately threw it back. The man said, "Mom, why did you do that?" His mother replied, "I don't know, to me it wasn't fresh."

My mother is also a stickler for freshness. She has even gone as far as to make her own sausages. She'll get casing from the pork store, coarsely grind a piece of fresh pork, and add her seasoning of fennel, oregano, pepper, parsley and sometimes grated cheese. Using a short, fat funnel, she miraculously makes sausages, twisting them into lengths so they're just like the sausages you buy from the butcher. However, hers are far superior, and are so good it pays to make more than you need and freeze half. You can make them into simple patties if you don't want to bother with the casings or buy a special sausage-stuffing funnel.

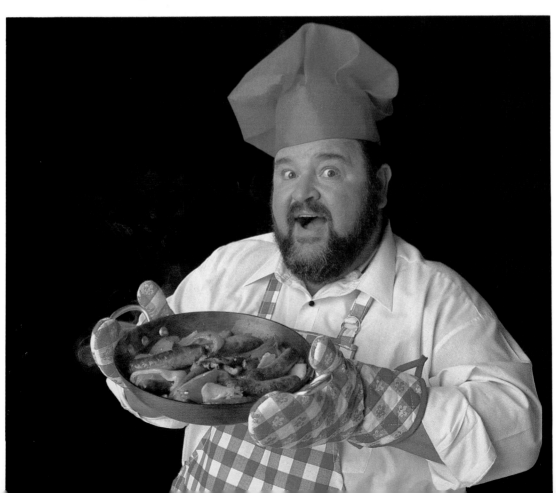

6 *pounds fresh, ground lean pork*
2 *tablespoons fennel*
1 *tablespoon pepper*
4 *tablespoons chopped fresh parsley*
6 *leaves fresh basil, chopped*
1 *teaspoon oregano*
1 *cup grated cheese (optional)*
4 *yards sausage casing*
  sausage funnel

Place all ingredients in a large mixing bowl. Mix well.

Push sausage casing onto funnel. Make a knot at the end and push meat through funnel with your thumb until the casing is all filled. Twist into links. Repeat until all the meat is gone.

Use immediately, or freeze some and refrigerate the rest, as these are perishable.

Gently brown in hot oil and then cook slowly in your spaghetti sauce. I think you'll find the taste incomparable.

Note: A good thing about homemade sausage is that you control the fat content. You can even make sausages out of chopped beef, veal, or turkey meat.

MAKES 30–35 SAUSAGES.

DOM'S MOM'S MEATBALLS

For as long as I can remember, my mother has never worn makeup. Also, she simply combs her hair straight back in a bun. Can you believe that when I was a child, I thought that bun was filled with meatballs? Good old Mom.

2 *pounds ground chuck*
½ *pound ground pork*
2 *cups Italian-flavored bread crumbs*
4 *eggs*
1 *cup milk*
1 *cup fresh parsley, chopped*

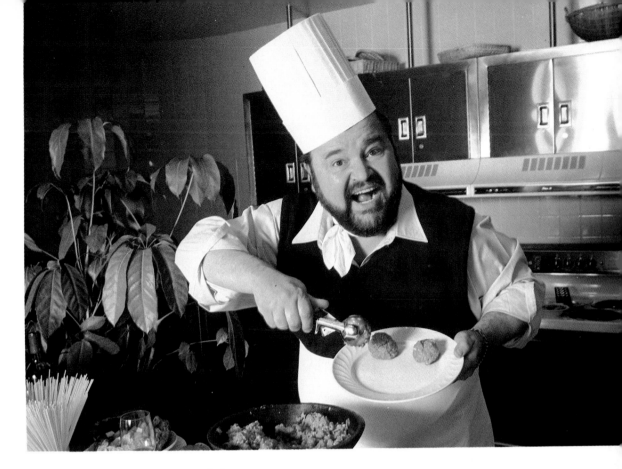

½ cup grated cheese
1 tablespoon olive oil
2 garlic cloves, chopped very fine
1 onion, minced
½ cup pignoli (pine nuts) (optional)

Place all ingredients in a large bowl and mix thoroughly. Let stand ½ hour. Shape into medium-size meatballs. Fry gently in olive oil until lightly browned, or place on foil on a cookie sheet and bake for ½ hour at 350 degrees. Gently place in your own hot spaghetti sauce and cook on medium-low heat for 1 hour.

P.S. What I like to do is quadruple the recipe (you'll have about 100 meatballs) and then place the meatballs on large Teflon baking pans. After they're baked and cooled, I put twenty at a time in large Ziploc bags and pop them in the freezer. Then they're ready, willing, and able *anytime!*

SERVES 10, 2 MEATBALLS PER PERSON.

DOM'S STEAMED DUMPLINGS

I think this recipe is absolutely splendid. I don't use the pork because of its fat content but I do use ground dark turkey meat and it's wonderful. You can steam the dumplings in a wok with a bamboo steamer.

Filling:

3	stalks of Chinese cabbage, chopped fine
1½	pounds ground pork butt—or better yet, ground turkey (dark meat)
1	onion, chopped fine
3	tablespoons soy sauce
1	teaspoon sugar
1	can bamboo shoots, drained, chopped fine
1	can water chestnuts, drained, chopped fine
1	tablespoon cornstarch
1	egg
	circle-shaped wonton wrappers
	or
	flour tortillas

Combine all the filling ingredients. Place 1 teaspoon of mixture in each wonton wrapper, pleat the sides in a circle, leaving the top open. Arrange dumplings on oiled bamboo steam rack in the wok, to which a little water has been added. Cover wok and steam for 15 minutes.

Or improvise—

Place ½ cup of filling mixture in the center of a flour tortilla. Roll halfway, tuck in sides, and roll all the way, ending up with seam on the bottom. Wrap individually in tinfoil and bake in 300-degree oven for 30 minutes.

Serve immediately with soy sauce and hot mustard, or Chinese Chicken Salad Dressing (page 54) on the side.

SERVES 6–8.

Note: Instead of chopping by hand, you can use a food processor for all the ingredients except the meat. Careful . . . don't overchop!

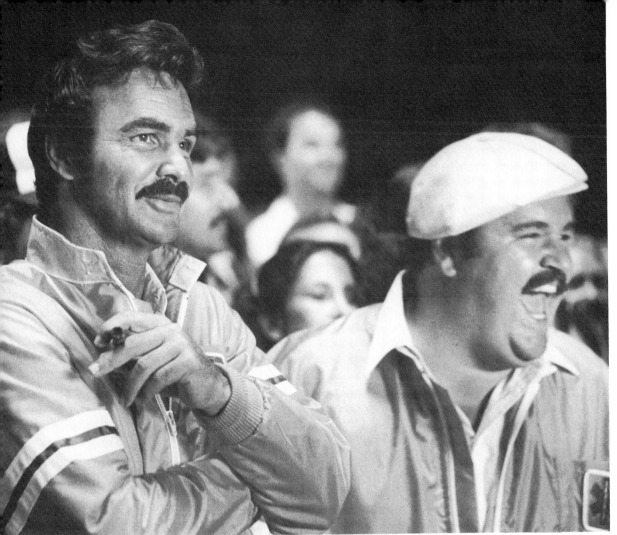

Me and my Hollywood look-alike in *Cannonball Run*.

BURT'S BEEF STEW

Burt Reynolds has been a really good friend of mine for many years, and I cherish my time with him. When we get together, we always eat, drink, and make merry.

Once a few of us were invited to Burt's for a party. And, lo and behold, Mr. Reynolds, Mr. Stud, Mr. Sex Symbol, announced that *he* had cooked dinner! Now I have known Burt for a long time and he does many things, and he does them very well, but he never cooked before, you know what I mean? We sat down to a candlelight dinner and Burt's *delicious* beef stew. I mean, can you imagine, my best buddy was not only cooking with gas in his bedroom, but was also holding his own in the kitchen!

3	*slices bacon, cut in small pieces*
4	*tablespoons flour*
¼	*teaspoon pepper*
2	*pounds lean beef (I like chuck) cut in chunks*
1	*large onion, chopped*
2	*cloves garlic, minced*
1	*28-oz. can tomato sauce*
1	*cup beef broth*
1	*cup dry red wine*
1	*bay leaf (optional)*
1	*pinch thyme*
4	*carrots, cut up coarsely*
2	*stalks celery, cut up coarsely*
4	*large potatoes, peeled and cut in 4 pieces each*

10–12 mushrooms, sliced

In a large pot or Dutch oven, cook bacon until light brown. Combine the flour and pepper in a bowl, dip the meat in the flour mixture to coat completely. Brown in bacon fat, turning often. Add a little vegetable oil if needed. Add onion and garlic and brown them a little. Add tomato sauce, broth, wine, bay leaf, and thyme. Cover and cook slowly for about 1½ hours. Add carrots, celery, then potatoes and mushrooms. Cook, covered, another ½ hour, or until vegetables are tender.

Serve with hot Italian bread, a large salad, fine wine, and good friends.

SERVES 1 MAN AND 3 OR 4 FRIENDLY LADIES. *Atta Boy, Burt!*

MAMMA'S VEAL MARSALA
"Fit for a King"

I worked with Frank Sinatra on "The Dean Martin Show" and again
on *Cannonball Run II*. He is a very special man, and I got an
enormous kick out of watching him and Dean work together. They
love each other so much, it kind of reminds me of the relationship I
have with Burt Reynolds . . . we're friends on and off the screen.
Frank's crazy about Italian food and he loves veal. So maybe if you
invite "The King" for dinner and present him with one of these veal
dishes, who knows? He might sing for his supper!

1   *pound boneless veal cut thin for scaloppine*
3   *tablespoons flour seasoned with pepper*
4   *tablespoons butter*
½   *pound fresh mushrooms, sliced*
2   *tablespoons beef bouillon*
½   *cup Marsala*
    fresh parsley for garnish

The King and I.

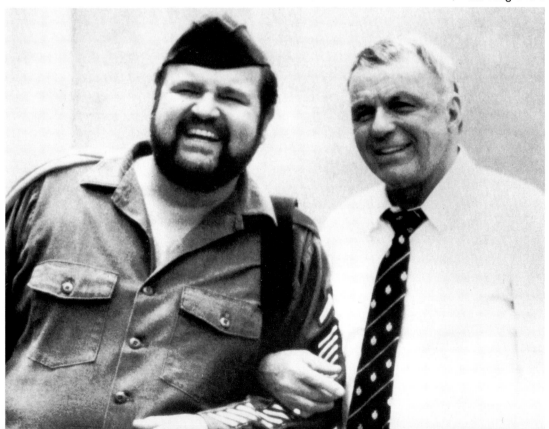

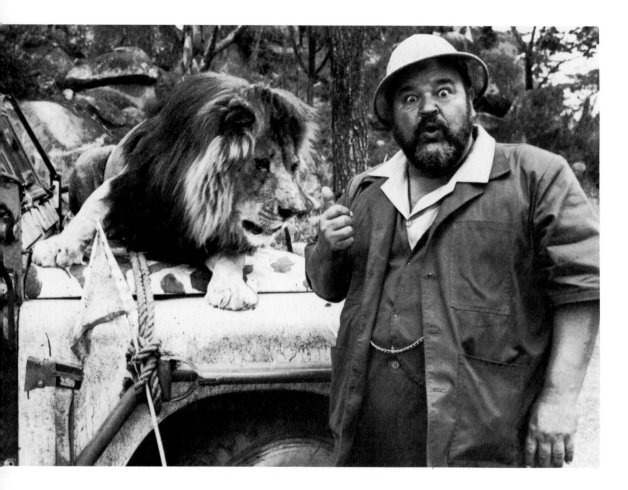

Put the veal between 2 pieces of wax paper and pound thin. Cut veal into serving pieces and coat each piece with flour. Heat butter in skillet until it sizzles, add the veal, and cook over high heat till browned on both sides. Add sliced mushrooms and sauté briefly. Add beef bouillon and Marsala, swoosh everything around in the pan and cook 1 minute longer. Arrange veal on a hot serving platter, pour pan juices over, and garnish with fresh parsley sprigs.

Variation: For the veal, substitute chicken breasts, sliced into cutlets and pounded between 2 pieces of wax paper, and prepare exactly like the veal. It's much cheaper and very delicious. Lots of people can't tell the difference.

SERVES 4.

Mamma . . . Compulsive Cooker!

One Mother's Day a couple of years ago, Carol had this brilliant idea. We were going to invite all the families, take over Mildred Pierce's, a restaurant in New York City, which is owned by our special friend, Bruce Laffey, and celebrate a spectacular Mother's Day! There were going to be about fifty people, and the good part was that no one— least of all Mamma—was supposed to cook!

We planned the tables to be arranged in a big horseshoe so that Mamma DeLuise and Carol's mother, Mrs. Arata, were sitting at the head with their children and grandchildren sitting around them. The party dinner was to start with a salad and consommé, then breast of chicken, asparagus, baked potato, and my famous cake, Death by Chocolate. Everything was ready.

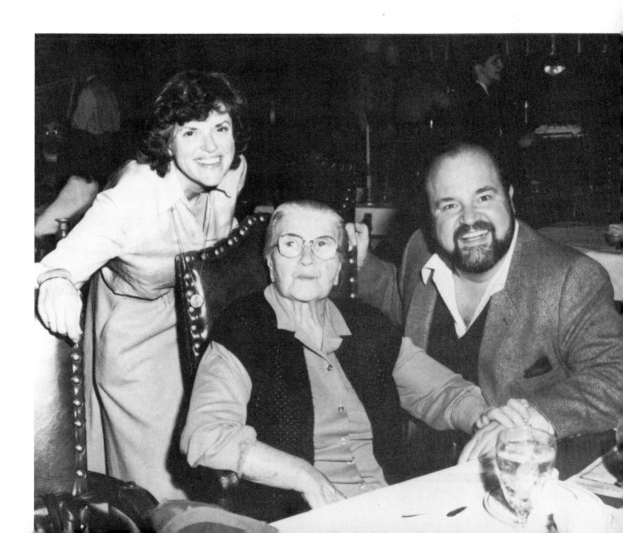

When Mother's Day came, my sister Anne went to Brooklyn to pick up Mamma at about 11:30 A.M. But when she got there, Mamma had prepared a huge tray of veal cutlets, homemade sausages with peppers and onions, and her famous birthday sponge cake with peaches, whipped cream and strawberries! What could Anne do? When they walked into the restaurant I couldn't believe my eyes. I said, "Mamma, you *cooked?*" She said, "It's just a taste." She then instructed the waiters to serve each person two pieces of veal, a sausage, and some peppers and onions. She also invited the waiters to have a taste while it was still hot. Talk about the best-laid plans! Bruce Laffey couldn't have been kinder. He embraced her, kissed her and thanked her for bringing these delicious dishes to his restaurant. You just can't keep a good cook down!

There were leftovers galore, and while we were all singing "M is for the million things she gave me," the very talented waiters were distributing them, beautifully wrapped in tinfoil and shaped like swans. Like fifty-two, to be exact. I think it was safe to presume everyone was going to be having chicken breasts the next day. Mamma's birthday cake was a big hit, and the never-ending laughter was mixed with groans from those who tried to taste both her cake and my own Death by Chocolate.

It's nice to think back on all these homecooked memories . . . "Put them all together they spell 'MOTHER,' the word that means the world to me." Right on, Mom! Happy Mother's Day!

MAMMA'S VEAL CUTLETS

1   *pound of veal cutlets, sliced very thin*
1   *cup flavored bread crumbs*
3 or 4 *large eggs*
         olive or peanut oil

First bread the veal cutlets with the crumbs and set aside. In a mixing bowl, place the eggs and beat very well. Dip breaded cutlets in egg mixture one by one, until crumbs are absorbed by mixture and cutlets are coated with this thick batter.

Heat 4 tablespoons of oil in a frying pan to medium hot. Fry the cutlets until golden brown on both sides. Remove from pan and place on paper towels to absorb excess oil. Use more oil as needed. Serve plain with lemon wedges.

Variation: Top each cutlet with tomato sauce and shredded mozzarella cheese and bake in 300-degree oven for 20 minutes, for Veal Parmesan.

SERVES 4–5.

VEAL PICCATA

Excellent for people who are in love—or if you are looking for a lasting relationship . . . start here!

1   *pound thinly cut veal scaloppine*
3   *tablespoons flour*
4   *tablespoons butter*
½   *pound fresh mushrooms, sliced*
½   *lemon*
½   *cup dry white wine*
       fresh parsley
       lemon slices

Cut veal slices into serving pieces, then coat each piece with flour. Heat butter in skillet until it sizzles. Add veal and cook over high heat until lightly browned on both sides. Add sliced mushrooms and sauté until brown.

Squeeze lemon over veal in pan, then add wine, swoosh everything around in pan, and cook 1 minute more.

Arrange veal on serving platter, garnish with parsley sprigs and round lemon slices.

SERVES 4.

Serve linguine with oil and garlic with this type of veal.

Reminder: Chicken breasts cut thin and pounded even thinner between wax paper are a great veal substitute.

STUFFED BREAST OF VEAL

One my of favorites—served with oven-baked potatoes, onions, and carrots. *Wow!*

1 *breast of veal (about 3 pounds)*
   a little olive oil
1 *cup ricotta cheese*
1 *egg, slightly beaten*
1 *10-oz. package of chopped spinach, defrosted and drained*
1 *onion, chopped*
¼ *teaspoon nutmeg*
   salt and pepper to taste

Preheat oven to 350 degrees. Make a slit (pocket) in the veal if this has not already been done at the market. Lightly coat with olive oil. Combine cheese, egg, spinach, onion and spices, and stuff into veal pocket. Place in a roasting pan and bake for about 1½ hours (30 minutes per pound).

Alternative: Replace this stuffing with your own favorite stuffing.

SERVES 4.

Note: This dish is very inexpensive to make, and very tasty. So be brave and try it!

DINAH'S MOUSSAKA

Dinah Shore is an incredibly talented person. She'll dazzle you on the tennis court or at golf, and she sings great too! I'm really crazy about this lady.

I've been to a couple of Dinah's dinner parties and everything she ever served was delicious. But there is one dish that Dinah Shore makes (and I have had it in Yugoslavia, Greece, and even New York City) that no one, I mean no one, makes as good as *Someone's in the Kitchen with Dinah*. In fact, I called Dinah up and asked if I could please put her incredible Moussaka recipe in my own cookbook. She just blew me a kiss.

3   *medium-sized eggplants*
1   *cup butter*
3   *large onions, finely chopped*
2   *pounds lamb or beef, ground*
3   *tablespoons tomato paste*
½   *cup red wine*
½   *cup parsley, chopped*
¼   *teaspoon cinnamon*
     salt to taste
     black pepper to taste, freshly ground
6   *tablespoons flour*
1   *quart milk*
4   *eggs, beaten until frothy*
     nutmeg
2   *cups ricotta or cottage cheese*
1   *cup fine bread crumbs*
1   *cup Parmesan cheese, freshly grated*

Peel the eggplants and cut them into slices about ½ inch thick. Brown the slices quickly in 4 tablespoons of the butter. Set aside.

Heat 4 tablespoons of butter in the same skillet and sauté the onions until they are brown. Add the ground meat and cook 10 minutes.

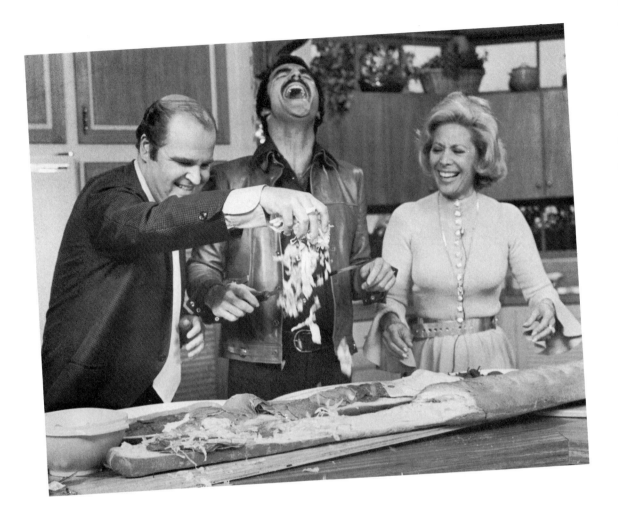

Combine the tomato paste with the wine, parsley, cinnamon, salt and pepper. Stir this mixture into the meat and simmer over low heat, stirring frequently, until all the liquid has been absorbed. Remove the mixture from the fire.

Preheat the oven to moderate (375 degrees).

Make a white sauce by melting 8 tablespoons of butter and blending in the flour, stirring with a wire whisk. Meanwhile, bring the milk to a boil and add it gradually to the butter-flour mixture, stirring constantly. When the mixture is thickened and smooth, remove it from the heat. Cool slightly and stir in the beaten eggs, nutmeg and ricotta.

Grease an 11-by-16-inch pan and sprinkle the bottom lightly with bread crumbs. Arrange alternate layers of eggplant and meat sauce in the pan, sprinkling each layer with Parmesan cheese and bread crumbs. Pour the ricotta sauce over the top and bake 1 hour, or until top is golden. Remove from the oven and let it cool a little before serving. Cut into squares and serve.

The flavor of this dish improves on standing 1 day. Reheat before serving.

SERVES 8–10. THAT'S WHAT DINAH SAYS, BUT I THINK IT FEEDS 16–18.

Seafood

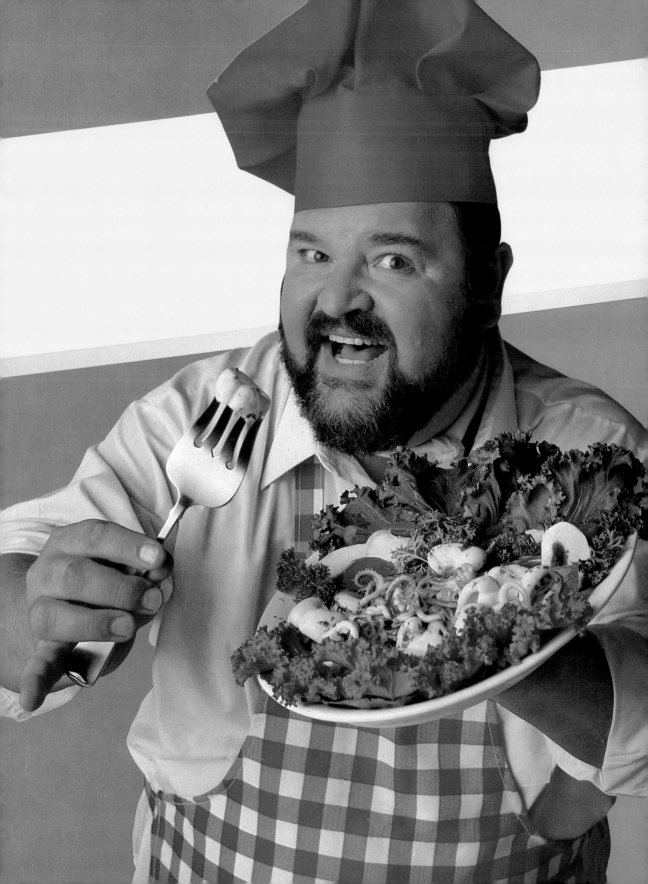

Two whole weeks before Christmas, my father would get a freshly cut Christmas tree and my brother Nick would decorate it with handmade and antique ornaments. My sister Anne was very meticulous about putting on the tinsel, and because I was the youngest, too small to reach the tree for decorating, I was in charge of the Nativity scene. I can remember slowly unwrapping those wonderful antique figures of the baby Jesus, Mary and Joseph, and the Three Wise Men. We even had a little sheep with real wool on it. It was my job to make sure there was a special Christmas-tree light to represent the star of Bethlehem and to see that there was a stable to hold all the little animals. I even built a manger with little pieces of old wood from our basement and filled it with some straw. I was very proud of my responsibility and was sure I had created the best Nativity scene ever. Then one year, oh, God, I must have been about seven years old . . . I shudder to think of it . . . I noticed that baby Jesus was a little dirty and decided to give him a bath. So I took baby Jesus to the sink and began to wash him, gently scrubbing him all over with a little Brillo, then rinsed him off. It was only as I was

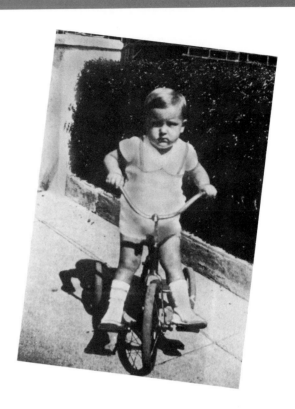

drying him that I suddenly noticed baby Jesus had no face! I was horrified as I looked closer and realized that I had scrubbed it off! I thought to myself, "Oh, Jesus, where's Your face? Now I'll never go to heaven!" I didn't know how I'd done what I'd done, but I was sure this sin was a "mortal." I remember crying and apologizing again and again to my mother, who was very understanding. It wasn't long before she brought home a brand-new baby Jesus, who, as far as I was concerned, could get as dirty as He wanted!

Christmas time created a bevy of unique foods. The Italians have a tradition on Christmas Eve to eat all different kinds of fish . . . shrimp, calamari (squid), baccalà (cod), polpi (octopus), sole, lobster. Christmas was indeed joyful, not only because of the food, but because it brought the whole family to the table, where there was a warm, safe, wonderful feeling of togetherness.

Let's Make Friends with Calamari

There's a great pasta restaurant in New York called Prego. The owner, Michael Cabot, has a terrific selection of lots of different pastas, but I'm very partial to the calamari sauce. In fact, calamari is one of my favorite foods with pasta, or in a cold salad. Prego's chef, Alfredo Baretta, does incredible things with calamari. It's always white and tender, always delicious. One night I sat with Alfredo and picked his brain about his technique, which he was gracious enough to share with me:

Clean and prepare calamari, removing eyes, ink sac and internal quill. Cut into rings and cut tentacles into pieces. Drop in boiling water in which you have placed a small piece of carrot, some onion, celery and ½ cup of white wine. Boil for three minutes until the calamari are plump, white and tender. Drain in colander.

This method is superb. However, if you're making a lot of calamari at once, it may take as long as 20 minutes to become tender. You might also be interested to know that a more traditional way of cooking calamari is to bread it, then deep-fry it. I prefer Alfredo's recipe because the calamari are *always* tender.

SALAD OF THE SEA

1 pound of squid, prepared as above, and chilled
1 pound cooked shrimp
   fresh parsley
   fresh basil
1 small onion, minced
1 3-oz. jar capers (drained)
4 celery stalks (chopped into small pieces)
4 tablespoons olive oil
2 tablespoons vinegar
2 tablespoons lemon juice
   Lettuce

Combine seafood, parsley, basil, onion, capers, and chopped celery. Gently toss with olive oil, vinegar and lemon juice. Serve on a bed of lettuce.

A very light Chinese vinegar works great on this salad too.

Note: When cooking shrimp, remember they cook fast. You can drop the shrimp in boiling water and as soon as they turn pink they are done. Or place them in your steamer and let them gently cook with steam. When they are pink, they are done and deliciously tender. Don't overcook your shrimp! Please!

SERVES 4–6.

STUFFED CALAMARI

2   pounds fresh calamari
1   garlic clove, sliced
2   tablespoons olive oil
2–3 cups crushed fresh tomatoes or
2   28-oz. cans crushed tomatoes

Clean and prepare calamari, removing eyes, ink sac and internal quill. Set aside. In a saucepan, combine garlic, olive oil, and tomatoes, and simmer ½ hour.

2 cups seasoned bread crumbs
1 cup grated cheese
1 tablespoon fresh parsley, chopped
4 leaves fresh basil
3 eggs
  pepper to taste

Mix all ingredients together until well blended. Using a sausage funnel, fill each calamari about ⅔ full (or use a small spoon to fill) and add calamari to above sauce. Simmer, covered, on low for 25 minutes or more, until tender.

This is delicious served with your favorite pasta.

SERVES 6.

BAKED CLAMS

Carol and I had a house on Fire Island, where our family could walk out of our front door, wade into the water and come back with dozens of fresh clams. I, therefore, spent the summer making baked clams. I couldn't make them fast enough. People ate them like popcorn! Opening them was a problem though, so, thank goodness, our neighbor, an eighty-seven-year-old lady, told me about the freezer trick.

2   *dozen clams*
8   *tablespoons olive oil*
10 *garlic cloves, minced*
1   *cup flavored bread crumbs*
1   *tablespoon oregano*
    olive oil
    lemon wedges

Place clams in freezer for 15 to 20 minutes to stun them. You'll see when you go to open them that they open easily. Save the juice and loosen each clam, leaving it in its bottom shell.

In a saucepan, heat the minced garlic gently until golden brown. Spoon a very little on each clam and mix the remainder with the bread crumbs, which you generously sprinkle to cover the clams in their shells. Sprinkle with oregano and a few more drops of olive oil.

Put them in a baking dish and then in a preheated 375-degree oven for 25 minutes.

Serve hot with plenty of lemon wedges and hot bread.

Fabulous!

SERVES 1–24 PEOPLE.

MAMMA'S MUSSELS

These mussels are so terrific, it is dangerous to ask anyone for a taste —they tend to snap: the people, not the mussels!

2 *tablespoons olive oil*
2 *tablespoons butter*
3 *garlic cloves, minced*
1 *small onion, minced*
2 *tablespoons chopped parsley*
4 *basil leaves, chopped*
¼ *teaspoon oregano*
   pepper
36 *fresh mussels, scrubbed and scraped clean*
1 *cup dry white wine*

In a deep saucepan, place the oil, butter, garlic, onion, parsley, basil, oregano and pepper. Stir and heat gently for 10 minutes. Then add mussels and wine. Cover saucepan, turn up heat until it boils, and then let simmer for 8 minutes, or until shells open.

Everyone gets a big bowl of the mussels and this lovely juice. With lemon wedges, it's wonderful.

SERVES 4–6.

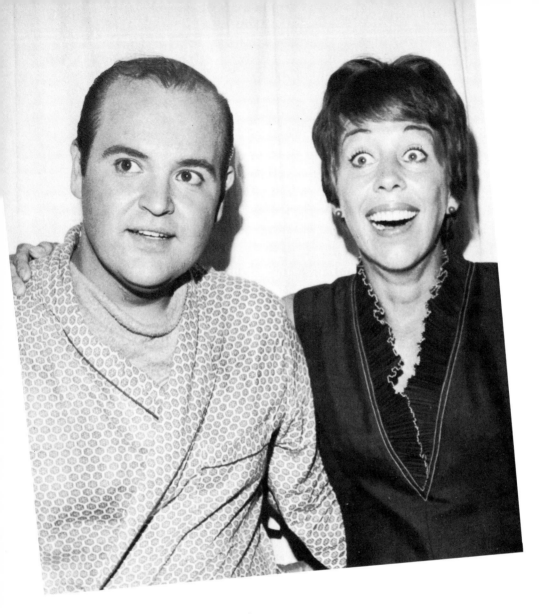

CAROL BURNETT'S SCAMPI

I've known Carol Burnett since 1964 when we were both involved in a television show called "The Entertainers." Carol is so much of a workaholic that when she was doing her television show, she gave exercise classes during her lunch hour. So naturally, when you go to Carol's house for dinner, you invariably end up playing a game that involves running and jumping and moving about. In other words, she is a fun high-energy lady. She also loves scampi, and here's a dish I named after her.

2   *tablespoons olive oil*
2   *tablespoons melted butter*
¼   *cup lemon juice*
    pepper to taste
3   *tablespoons shallots, finely minced*
3   *garlic cloves, finely minced*
2   *pounds jumbo shrimp or prawns, shelled and deveined*
    lemon slices and parsley for garnish

Combine olive oil, melted butter, lemon juice, pepper, shallots, and garlic in a shallow baking dish. Add shrimp and turn several times to coat thoroughly.

Place the dish of shrimp in a preheated broiler about 4 inches from the heat for about 2 minutes, turn and broil on the other side for 1 minute more. Don't overcook. Arrange on a serving platter and pour remaining sauce over the shrimp. Garnish with lemon and sprinkle with parsley, serve hot and stand back!

SERVES 6–8.

They'll fight over this!

MAMMA'S ITALIAN FISH STEW

My papa just loved this dish. As it was served he would merely sit and smile. Papa was a quiet man . . . until he began eating! Folks, one of the noisiest meals ever, and one of Mamma's most famous creations.

4   *tablespoons olive oil*
3   *garlic cloves, minced*
1   *onion, chopped*
1   *large tomato, diced*
1   *green pepper, chopped*
1   *red pepper, chopped*
1   *celery stalk, chopped*
1   *cup dry white wine*
2   *28-oz. cans crushed tomatoes*
1   *8-oz. bottle clam juice*
½   *pound calamari (squid), skinned, cleaned and cut into small pieces*
½   *pound cod fillet or red snapper, in 1½-inch pieces pepper to taste*
½   *teaspoon oregano*
¼   *teaspoon thyme*
½   *pound shrimp, shelled and deveined*
½   *pound scallops*
6   *clams, well scrubbed*

In a large kettle, heat the oil. Add the garlic, onion, tomato, peppers, and celery, and sauté lightly. Add the white wine, crushed tomatoes, and clam juice, and bring to a boil. Lower heat to a simmer, throw in the squid, and cook 3 minutes. Add the cod and the red snapper, and simmer for about 10 minutes (add a little water at your own discretion, but the liquid should be thick). Season with pepper, oregano and thyme. At this point, add the shrimp, scallops and clams and cook for another 5 minutes.

Serve in large bowls with plenty of hot Italian bread and BIG napkins.

SERVES 6.

DOM'S STUFFED SOLE

"Sole food" Dom style—lovely with white wine, a candle, friends, and mashed potatoes . . . not necessarily in that order.

5   *tablespoons olive oil*
2   *tablespoons lemon juice*
2   *tablespoons chopped chives*
3   *garlic cloves, minced*
6   *fillets of sole*
12 *mushrooms, sliced*
½   *cup pignoli (pine nuts) or blanched almonds*
2   *cups fresh spinach, chopped*
3   *green onions, chopped*
    parsley and lemon slices for garnish

In a bowl, combine 3 tablespoons oil, lemon juice, chives, and garlic. Wash fish and pat dry. Place in baking dish and pour oil mixture over fish.

Heat remaining oil in a skillet and sauté mushrooms and nuts. Add spinach and onions. Cook until spinach is soft and remove from flame.

Remove fish from marinade and stuff with mushroom mixture. Roll up and arrange in baking dish, seam side down. Spoon marinade over fish.

Bake at 400 degrees for 15 minutes. Garnish with parsley and lemon slices.

SERVES 6.

Variation: A fast and easy way to do this is to omit the mushroom-spinach stuffing and use a Stouffer's frozen spinach soufflé to stuff the fish.

BOUILLABAISSE

Norman and Frances Lear had a dinner party and they served "a one-dish meal called Bouillabaisse." I never heard so much praise for fish soup . . . wowwee! It's formidáble!

Fish Stock:

1–2	*pounds fish heads and bones of white-fleshed fish*	1	*bay leaf*
2	*garlic cloves, chopped*	1	*tomato, quartered*
1	*small onion, quartered*	1	*teaspoon oregano*
1	*celery stalk, sliced*	1	*parsley sprig*
4	*peppercorns*		*juice of ½ lemon*

Simmer above ingredients in 2 to 3 quarts of water for about 2 hours. Add water as needed. Strain the fish stock into a large kettle. Discard fish heads, bones, and bits of remaining vegetables.

Bouillabaisse:

2–3	*quarts fish stock*		*white pepper*
4	*8-oz. bottles clam juice*	2	*dashes hot pepper sauce*
1	*12-oz. bottle beer*	4	*4-ounce halibut fillets,*
2	*carrots, sliced*		*½ inch thick*
4	*celery stalks, sliced*	4	*8-ounce lobster tails,*
4	*garlic cloves, minced*		*cut in half*
1	*leek, diced*	8–12	*medium shrimp, shelled*
4–8	*saffron threads*		*and deveined*
1	*tablespoon cornstarch*	12–16	*scallops*
2	*cups dry white wine*	8–12	*clams, well scrubbed*

To the large kettle of fish stock, add the clam juice, beer, carrots, celery, garlic, leek, and saffron. Bring to a boil, reduce heat, and simmer until carrots are tender-crisp. Combine cornstarch with 1 cup wine and stir into simmering kettle. Simmer 5 minutes and season to taste with pepper and hot pepper sauce. Add halibut, lobster tails, shrimp, scallops and clams. Add the remaining 1 cup wine. Bring to a boil for 8–10 minutes, or until seafood is done and all the clams are open.

Serve in large bowls with generous amounts of the liquid. This is wonderful served with garlic toast or hot, crispy French bread and white wine.

SERVES 6–8.

CHEF PAUL PRUDHOMME'S BLACKENED REDFISH

I had heard about Paul Prudhomme and his Blackened Redfish for a long time. So when I was in New Orleans I decided to dress up like him, go to his restaurant, "K-Paul's," and call him an imposter in front of all his customers. When he found out I was coming, he called the TV people, and our famous "confrontation" is now immortalized on tape!

If you don't have a commercial hood vent over your stove, this dish may smoke you out of the kitchen, but it's worth it! You can also cook it outdoors on a grill.

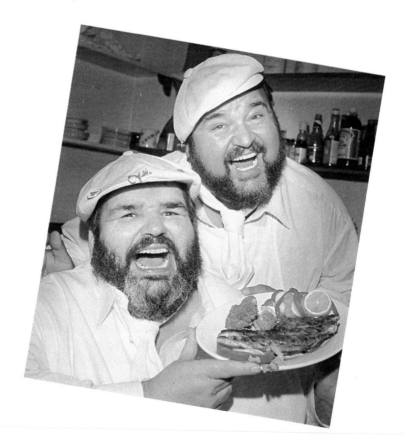

3   sticks unsalted butter, melted in a skillet

Seasoning Mix:
(Or substitute Chef Prudhomme's Blackened Redfish Magic . . .
That's what I use, folks!)
1   teaspoon sweet paprika
2½ teaspoons salt . . . Oh, Paul, how could you!
1   teaspoon onion powder
1   teaspoon garlic powder
1   teaspoon ground red pepper (preferably Cayenne)
¾   teaspoon white pepper
¾   teaspoon black pepper
½   teaspoon dried thyme leaves
½   teaspoon dried oregano leaves

6   8–10-oz. fish fillets (preferably redfish, pompano or tilefish), cut
about ½-inch thick

Note: Redfish and pompano are ideal for this dish. If tilefish is used, you may have to split the fillets in half horizontally to have the proper thickness. If you can't get any of these fish, salmon steaks or red snapper fillets can be substituted. In any case, the fillets or steaks must not be more than ¾ inch thick.

Heat a large *cast iron* skillet over very high heat until it is beyond the smoking stage and you see the skillet bottom start to turn ashen—at least 10 minutes.

Meanwhile, pour 2 tablespoons melted butter in each of 6 small ramekins; set aside and keep warm. Reserve the remaining butter in its skillet. Heat the serving plates in a 250-degree oven.

Thoroughly combine the seasoning-mix ingredients in a small bowl. Dip each fillet in the reserved melted butter so that both sides are well coated; then sprinkle the seasoning mix generously and evenly on both sides of the fillets, patting it in by hand. Place in the hot cast-iron skillet and pour 1 teaspoon melted butter on top of each fillet (be careful, as the butter may flame up). Cook uncovered over high heat until the underside looks charred, about 2 minutes (the time will vary according to the fillet's thickness and the heat of the skillet). Turn the fish over and pour 1 teaspoon more butter on top; cook until fish is done, about 2 minutes more. Repeat with remaining fillets. Serve each fillet while piping hot.

To serve, place 1 fillet and a ramekin of butter on each heated serving plate.

SERVES 6.

LOAVES AND FISHES

Kevin Carlisle and I were in summer stock together in Cleveland, Ohio, when we were eighteen years old. He is now a choreographer who works with Barry Manilow, Dionne Warwick and Melissa Manchester. We were invited to Kevin's house for a Hollywood party and he served this wonderful dish. People flipped over it. When the insides were finished they gobbled up the bread on the outside leaving Kevin with nothing but the pan he served it in!

1	*can cream of mushroom soup (trust me)*
2	*8-oz. packages cream cheese*
1	*jar of Ortega green chili salsa*
6–8	*mushrooms, sliced thin*
2	*cups fresh crab meat*
1	*Sheepherder's bread (or a good hard-crusted round loaf)*

In a saucepan place soup and cream cheese and stir gently over low heat until cream cheese is softened. Add Ortega sauce, cook another 10 minutes.

Take Sheepherder's bread (round), cut off top, hollow out bread, and add mushrooms and crab meat. Then add contents of saucepan. Stir gently, replace top and heat bread in 350-degree oven for 35 minutes. Serve with extra pieces of hot bread.

Trust me! MMMMM . . . good!

SERVES 1 HUNGRY FISHERMAN FOR DINNER, OR 10–15 AS HORS D'OEUVRES.

Bread

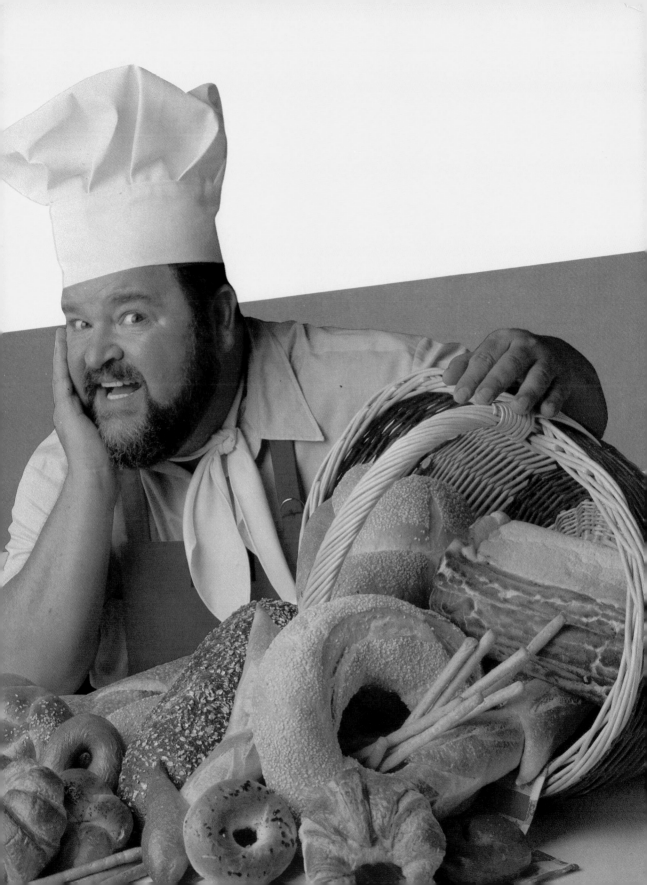

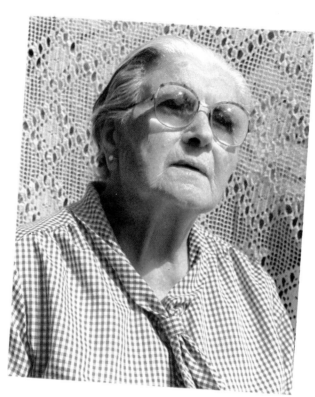

My family's Easter holiday had more baking than any other time. As Catholics, we had just finished Lent and looked forward to Good Friday and Easter, when we would remember the Ascension of Christ. So in our house the dough was rising all the time. My mother would spend days making sweet Papoose Bread, Easter Grain Pie (Pizza Grana), Strufoli with melted honey sprinkled with confetti, and her special Braided Egg Bread. It was like a giant pretzel calling to me! While the rest of America was experiencing bunny rabbits and colored eggs, incredible shapes and wonderful tastes were coming out of my mother's oven faster than you can say, "He has risen."

At noon on Easter Sunday the church bells across the street would ring so the windows would tremble! The memory of this joyous sound —along with all the other neighborhood church bells ringing—still brings tears to my eyes. It was at that precise moment that Mamma led the ritual which would truly begin the Easter celebration for our family. There was a marble threshold in our house and under it was a steam pipe that made it warm. When she heard the bells, my mother would immediately bend down to kiss this threshold, then the rest of us would do the same. We embraced—and the feasting began! Here are some of the breads I remember from that happy time, and some other favorites as well.

MAMMA'S EASTER PAPOOSE BREAD

Every Easter my mother sends our family in Los Angeles a package from Brooklyn: her traditional Easter papooses, one for each of us. All the DeLuises love them. By the way, it is called "papoose" because the shape of the bread looks very much like a baby wrapped in a blanket.

¼	cup lukewarm water
1	teaspoon plus ½ cup sugar
1	package active dry yeast
1	cup scalded milk
	pinch of salt
⅓	cup butter
2	eggs, beaten
3½	cups unsifted flour
1	egg, beaten well with
1	teaspoon water
6	eggs in their shells
	confetti sprinkles

Combine water, 1 teaspoon sugar, and yeast in a small bowl and let stand 5 minutes. In a large bowl, combine milk, salt, butter, eggs, and remaining ½ cup sugar. Add about half the flour and beat until smooth. Stir in yeast mixture.

Slowly add the remaining flour to form a stiff dough (add more flour if needed), turn out on a floured board and knead until smooth. Place in a greased bowl, cover and let rise in a warm place until doubled.

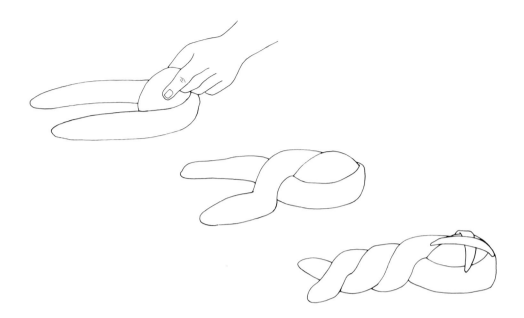

Punch down the dough, return to the floured board and divide into 6 pieces. Roll each piece to form a 1-inch-thick rope and make a U-shape. Place an egg on the inside of each "U," twist the lengths, forming a fishtail at the bottom. Brush with beaten egg mixture, sprinkle with confetti and place on a greased baking sheet.

Cover and let rise until double in size. Bake at 350 degrees until brown—about 35 minutes. Cool on a rack for about 10 minutes.

MAKES 6 PAPOOSE BREADS.

Note A: Eggs do not need to be cooked. They become hard during the baking process.

Note B: You can use eggs tinted with nontoxic dye.

MAMMA'S BRAIDED EGG BREAD

All nationalities seem to have an equivalent of this bread . . . like a Jewish challah. No matter what the nationality, it's all the same: great toasted, with a little butter and jam.

1   *package active dry yeast*
1¼   *cups warm water*
2   *teaspoons sugar*
2   *teaspoons salad oil*
4½   *cups all-purpose flour*
2   *eggs*
1   *egg yolk, beaten with 1 teaspoon water*
3   *tablespoons sesame seeds*

In a large mixing bowl, sprinkle yeast over ¼ cup of the warm water. Let stand until soft (about 5 minutes). Add remaining 1 cup of warm water, sugar, and oil.

Mix in 3 cups of the flour, and beat at medium speed until smooth and elastic (about 5 minutes). You can also do this by hand. Beat in eggs, one at a time, and gradually stir in about 1½ cups flour to make a soft dough.

Turn dough out onto a floured board and knead until dough is smooth and satiny and small bubbles form just under the surface. Add more flour if dough becomes sticky.

Turn dough into a greased bowl. Cover and let rise in a warm place until doubled . . . about 1 hour. Punch dough down, cover again, and let rise until doubled . . . about 45 minutes. Punch down and divide into 3 equal portions.

On a lightly floured board, roll each portion into an 18-inch strand. Place the 3 strands on a greased baking sheet and braid, pinching the ends together. Let rise until doubled . . . about 45 minutes. Brush with egg-yolk mixture and sprinkle with sesame seeds. Bake at 375 degrees for about 45 minutes or until crust is golden brown and loaf sounds hollow when tapped.

MAKES 1 LOAF.

MOM'S SAUSAGE BREAD

This is one bread you can really get your teeth into. But be careful because it bites back!

1   *package active dry yeast*
¼   *cup warm water*
1   *cup warm milk*
1   *tablespoon sugar*
2   *tablespoons olive oil*
3¼ *cups all-purpose flour*
½   *cup whole-wheat flour*
1   *pound sweet Italian sausages*
1   *medium onion, chopped*
1   *egg, beaten with 1 teaspoon water*

Sprinkle yeast over warm water in large bowl. Let stand until soft (about 5 minutes). Stir in milk, sugar, and 1 tablespoon of the oil.

Add 2½ cups of the flour. Mix to blend, then beat at medium speed until smooth and elastic (about 5 minutes). You can also beat by hand. Stir in whole-wheat flour and about ¼ cup more of the all-purpose flour to make a stiff dough.

Turn dough out onto a lightly floured board. Knead until dough is smooth and satiny and small bubbles form just under the surface (about 15 minutes). Add more flour if dough becomes sticky.

Turn dough into a greased bowl. Cover and let rise in a warm place until doubled—about 1 hour. While dough is rising, remove sausage meat from casing and crumble into a frying pan. Add chopped onion and brown the sausage meat and onion lightly, over medium heat, stirring often. Remove meat and onion and let them cool and drain on paper towels.

Punch dough down and form into a ½-inch-thick circle. Sprinkle sausage and onion over dough. Knead and fold lightly into dough. Shape into a ball and pat out to a mound about 8 inches in diameter.

Brush dough with the remaining tablespoon of oil and let rise for about 30 minutes. Brush with egg mixture. Bake at 375 degrees for about 30 minutes or until crust is golden brown and loaf sounds hollow when tapped.

MAKES 1 LOAF.

PUMPKIN BREAD IN A COFFEE CAN TELEPHONE

When I was an eight-year-old growing up in Brooklyn, I had a best friend named June Fucci. From my second-floor window to her second-floor window there was a clothesline which we'd use to send notes back and forth, or sometimes we would just sit and talk to each other out the window for hours. One day we each got a coffee can, put a hole in the bottom of it, and ran a long waxed string from can to can, tying a knot on the inside of each can. We ran the string from window to window and whispered into our coffee cans so that nobody could hear our secret conversations. Oh, the magic of it! We made our own telephone!

One day I couldn't find my "coffee can telephone" to call June. I asked Mamma if she had seen it anyplace, and she said, "Yes, it's in the oven." My dismay quickly disappeared, though, when I tasted the wonderful pumpkin bread she baked that day . . . in my coffee can telephone!

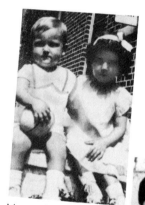

Me and Junie, as kids.

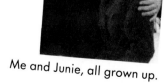

Me and Junie, all grown up.

¾	cup sugar
1	teaspoon brown sugar
½	cup oil or melted butter
2	eggs, beaten
½	teaspoon black walnut extract (or almond extract)
1¾	cups flour
1	teaspoon baking soda
1	teaspoon baking powder
½	teaspoon cinnamon
1	cup cooked pumpkin, mixed with ⅓ cup water (canned pumpkin is OK)
1	cup walnuts

Mix sugars and butter together and stir in beaten eggs. Add walnut extract. Sift flour, baking powder, baking soda, and cinnamon together. Alternate adding the sugar mixture and the pumpkin and nuts to the flour. Mix well after each addition.

Turn into 3 greased and floured 1-pound coffee cans. Bake at 350 degrees for 45 minutes or until a cake tester inserted in the center of the bread comes out clean. Cool 10 minutes, loosen the bread from the can by running a knife between the bread and the can. Open the bottom of the can with an opener and push the bread through the top of the can. *Voilà!*

MAKES 3 BREADS.

CHEESE AND ONION BREAD

After I had the first taste of my friend Sadie Ratliff's bread, I told her that I would keep her children (whom I love) if she didn't give me the recipe!

1½	*cups chopped onion*	1	*tablespoon baking powder*
2	*tablespoons butter*	¼	*cup butter*
1	*egg*	1	*cup shredded Cheddar cheese*
½	*cup sour cream*	⅔	*cup milk*
	pepper	3	*tablespoons fresh parsley,*
2	*cups flour*		*minced*

Sauté onion in 2 tablespoons butter until tender. In a bowl, combine onions with egg, sour cream, and pepper. Mix well. Set aside.

Add flour and baking powder to another bowl. Cut in ¼ cup butter until crumbly and fine. Stir in half the cheese. Add milk to make a soft dough. Pat dough into a buttered 9-inch-square pan. Spread sour-cream mixture on top.

Sprinkle with remaining cheese and parsley. Bake in oven at 425 degrees for 25 minutes. Cut into squares. Serve warm.

SERVES 8.

When I was fifteen years old, growing up in Brooklyn was enhanced by an occasional trip to the Big Apple—New York City. My best friend, Salvatore Orena, and I would see a movie and then take the BMT back to Brooklyn. One night Sal and I stayed out real late and were so tired coming home that we feel asleep on the subway and missed our stop. We woke up at the end of the line, Coney Island. So we took the next train back, desperately trying to stay awake. Naturally, the stop before we were supposed to get off we fell asleep again and woke up at the other end of the line, 42nd Street! But this time, when we got on the train, we asked the conductor to please wake us up so we could get off at the right stop. It worked.

So, it was 4:30 A.M. Saturday morning, as I was walking home, when the smell of freshly baked bread stopped me in my tracks in front of the bread store. I looked inside the store and saw the baker taking hot loaves of Italian bread out of the oven. Two minutes and 15 cents later I was happily juggling a steaming loaf of the hottest bread I ever tried to carry home. Talk about hot potatoes! By the time I got home at 4:45 A.M., a "midnight snack" seemed appropriate. I cut the

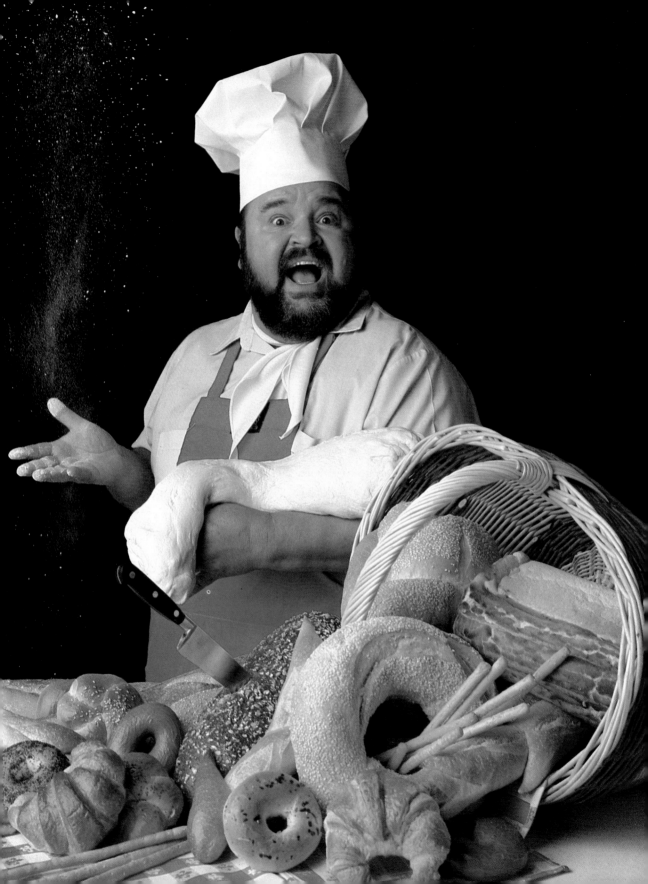

hot loaf in half and then split it lengthwise, adding slices of beefsteak tomato with a dribble of olive oil, and a little salt and pepper. I leaned over the kitchen sink and bit into one of the best tastes I can ever remember.

Years later when I told my friend Anne Bancroft about this, she was struck by the story. In fact, when she became homesick while in England filming *Young Winston,* she ordered from the room-service waiter at the very elegant Connaught Hotel a hot loaf of bread, some tomatoes and olive oil, which he served to her on a silver tray. Anne said it was just the taste she needed to remind her of her family in New York. I, however, think eating this sandwich over the kitchen sink is the most important part of the experience.

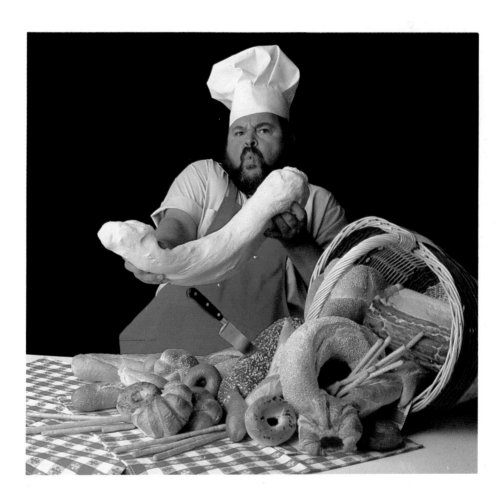

AUNT ROSE'S ZUCCHINI BREAD

My wife, Carol, has an Aunt Rose, a born cook, who makes the best zucchini bread ever. And now you can too. Here is her recipe:

3   *cups flour*
1½ *cups sugar*
1   *teaspoon cinnamon*
1   *pinch salt*
1   *teaspoon baking powder*
1   *teaspoon baking soda*
3   *cups shredded, unpeeled zucchini*
1   *cup raisins*
1   *cup nuts*
3   *eggs*
2   *teaspoons vanilla*
1   *cup oil*

In a large bowl, mix together the flour, sugar, cinnamon, salt, baking powder, baking soda, zucchini, raisins, and nuts. In another bowl, beat together the eggs, vanilla, and oil. Pour over flour mixture and stir until thoroughly mixed. Turn into 2 greased loaf pans. Bake at 350 degrees for approximately 1½ hours.

MAKES 2 LOAVES.

MARY DAURIO'S BEER BREAD

My niece, Mary, is like a child of God. She is one of the sweetest people I know and very easy to love. Wouldn't you know that her beer bread has only 3 ingredients and is very easy also! Her husband, Peter, is a great guy and a really fine cook, for a Canadian.

3 *cups self-rising flour*
1 *12-oz. can of beer*
2 *tablespoons sugar*

Mix ingredients and put into greased loaf pan. Don't overmix. Bake at 375 degrees for about 1 hour.

Options: You can cut down on the self-rising flour and add whole-wheat flour, bran flakes, rolled oats, nuts, and ½ cup raisins in any combination. For example, I use 1 cup white flour, 1 cup whole-wheat flour, ½ cup bran flakes and ½ cup rolled oats.

MAKES 1 LOAF.

PIZZA DOUGH

This dough is great for pizza, Mamma's Spinach Rolls, and calzone. The nice part of it is, you can freeze it until you are ready to use. Just thaw it out and let it rise to the occasion.

1 package dry yeast
1 cup warm water
3 cups flour
1 tablespoon olive oil

Dissolve the yeast in warm water. Place flour on a clean smooth surface in a mound with a well in the center. Add water-and-yeast mixture. Gather flour from the sides with a fork or fingertips. Working with hands, combine in a dough ball. Knead until soft and smooth (about 15 minutes). Add flour as necessary. Place in a large, oiled bowl. Cover and put in a warm spot until about double the size. Punch the dough down, cut in half and roll out on a floured board.

MAKES 2 TEN-INCH PIZZAS.

Note: Great with tomato sauce and cheese, and/or pepperoni, onion, peppers, anchovies, olives, etc., etc.

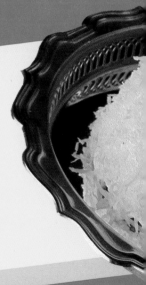

Desserts

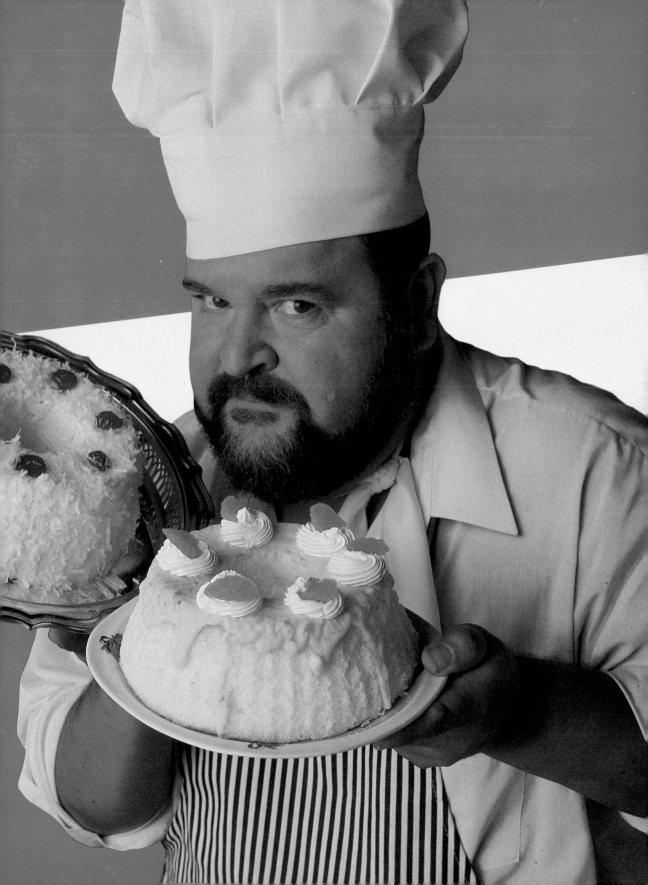

I must tell you that some of the desserts in this section are absolutely lethal: I've included some out-and-out chocolate and chocolate chip cakes that will devastate your children, friends, husbands, and lovers. I mean, you know, like Death by Chocolate, simply the best chocolate cake in the world! On the other hand, there are some marvelous recipes that your guests will only *think* are lethal, yet are anything but. I make a sugarless baked apple dish (page 231) for example, that is sensible and healthy but also tastes like heaven! Wherever your sweet tooth takes you, though, all of these recipes are, mmmm, *incredible!*

P.S. Folks, there is no recipe for fruitcake in this cookbook, because I don't think anybody really bakes them. I think people get them in the mail, keep them awhile, and then send them on to somebody else. Actually, there are only about 28 fruitcakes in the whole country. People just keep sending them back and forth to each other. So, if you want fruitcake, just wait till somebody mails you one, open it and eat it, but I can't be responsible for the consequences. You may be breaking up a whole chain of events. You are on your own!

MAMMA'S HAPPY BIRTHDAY, ANNIVERSARY, AND WEDDING CAKE

Happy Birthday to You
Happy Birthday to You
You're Gonna Get the Same Cake
No Matter What You Do

If you're three years old, or if you're eighty years old, my mother will make you exactly the same birthday cake. It may not taste like Death by Chocolate, but it's certainly the freshest, lightest, healthiest . . . and to my mind the most delicious cake in the world!

My mom is eighty-eight, God bless her, and she says, "For sixty-five years I have been making this cake. I never had any complaints and I never had any leftovers."

Note: Also good for anniversaries, weddings, and bar mitzvahs.

6 eggs, separated	wax paper
1 cup sugar	2 round 9-inch baking pans
1 teaspoon vanilla	electric beater and mixing bowl
2 heaping teaspoons baking powder	
1 cup flour	

Beat egg whites until foamy. Slowly add egg yolks to egg whites, one at a time. Then add sugar and vanilla. Add baking powder to flour and gradually add to the other ingredients and mix well.

Pour half the batter into each round pan, both of which have been lined with wax paper. Bake at 350 degrees for 15 to 20 minutes. Remove from pan, cool cakes on rack. Remove wax paper (it peels off easily).

Topping:
1   medium can crushed pineapple
1½ pints of heavy cream for whipping
3   teaspoons sugar
1   large can sliced peaches
12   strawberries, cut in half

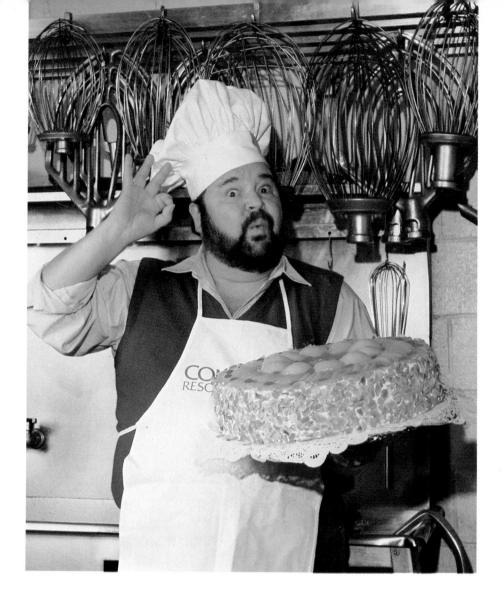

Whip cream with sugar until it peaks.

On serving dish, place 1st layer, on which you evenly spread crushed pineapple and 1 cup of whipped cream. Cover with 2nd layer and dribble peach juice evenly over top. Spread the rest of the whipped cream generously over top and sides of cake. Decorate top with sliced peaches and strawberries.

Alternative 1: Use strawberries in place of pineapple or peaches.

Alternative 2: Use Mamma's custard (page 216) on bottom layer and cover top with whipped cream.

YIELDS 2 CAKES: 1 FOR TOP AND 1 FOR BOTTOM LAYER. SERVES 8–10.

CRISPELLE

It wouldn't be Christmas without these traditional holiday taste treats!

1½ *cups flour*
1   *teaspoon baking powder*
2   *large eggs*
2   *egg yolks*
       vegetable oil
½   *cup honey*
       confetti (tiny candy dots)

Put flour on a pastry board, make a wide well in the center of it, and mix baking powder, eggs, and egg yolks into flour. Continue mixing until you have a solid mass. Then knead dough with your hands until it has a firm and smooth consistency.

Separate the dough into 3 portions and, with a rolling pin, roll the first portion out to about a ⅛-inch thickness. Sprinkle flour over sparingly to keep dough from sticking. Then, with pastry wheel, make 1-inch strips, fold them into pretzels, bows, or your favorite shape, and drop into 2 inches of vegetable oil at medium heat. If the dough comes to the top quickly, the oil is hot enough. When the shapes are golden brown, take them out and put them on paper towels to drain. Heat honey over low heat in a saucepan, then dribble it over the crispelle. Sprinkle the whole thing with confetti and arrange in a serving dish.

MAKES ABOUT 24.

Note: My favorite shape is to cut a 6-inch diamond, make a slit, and tuck the corners in and around the slit; then fry it.

STRUFOLI

Every nationality has its equivalent of these marvelous marble-sized balls of fried dough covered with honey and sprinkled with candy confetti. They also stay fresh forever and they freeze really well . . . that is, if there are any left over!

4   *eggs*
¼   *cup sugar*
1   *teaspoon vanilla*
1   *teaspoon cinnamon*
1   *tablespoon margarine*
2½   *cups flour*
½   *cup honey*
     vegetable oil
     confetti

In a large bowl, mix together eggs, sugar, vanilla, cinnamon and margarine. Add flour, 1 cup at a time. The last ½ cup of flour can be added if necessary to make a smooth dough. Let dough stay in bowl, covered with a dish, for ½ hour.

Roll out portions of dough. Cut dough into strips, rounded like pretzels, then cut in ½-inch pieces.

Heat about 2½ inches of oil in the bottom of a pan. Fry the pieces of dough, a handful at a time. If you can do this in a frying basket, it will be easier to take them out. Place pieces on paper towels to drain.

Heat honey until just under the boiling point. Place strufoli in a bowl and drizzle honey over them, gently tossing. Arrange on a large platter and sprinkle with confetti. (Shape into a mound on a large flat dish or into a wreath.)

MAKES ABOUT 150 LITTLE STRUFOLI.

MOM'S EASTER GRAIN PIE (PIZZA GRANA)

Mamma always makes this traditional pie for Easter. The textures of the grain and the taste of the ricotta intermingle to make nice in your mouth!

2½ *cups sifted flour*
2½ *cups sugar*
8   *eggs*
⅓   *cup shortening*
2   *teaspoons vanilla*
      grated rind of 1 lemon (yellow part only)
      grated rind of 1 orange (orange part only)
3   *pounds ricotta cheese*
1   *cup cooked wheat grain (wheat grain may be found in health food stores)*
½   *cup citron*

First make a piecrust by blending together flour and shortening. Add ½ cup sugar, 2 eggs, 1 teaspoon vanilla and orange and lemon rind. Blend well and roll flat on a floured cutting board. Place in a 10-by-13-inch-by-2-inch-deep baking pan and set aside.

To make filling, separate remaining 6 eggs and beat egg whites until they form soft peaks. Set aside.

Beat egg yolks well and add 1 teaspoon vanilla, ricotta cheese, 2 cups sugar, grain, and citron. Blend well and slowly fold in egg whites.

Carefully pour into piecrust and bake at 400 degrees for 10 minutes. Reduce heat to 350 degrees and bake 40 minutes more until light golden brown.

MAKES 1 LARGE 10-INCH PIE.

ZEPPOLI

On New Year's Eve, in some homes, zeppoli are filled with all kinds of things. They help make the coming year seem brighter! But . . . any time is zeppoli time! Go get 'em while they're hot!

1   *packet dry yeast*
1   *cup lukewarm water*
1½ *cups flour*
    safflower oil, for deep frying
    powdered sugar

Dissolve the yeast in ½ cup warm water. Put the remaining water in a large pan and add the flour all at once, beating vigorously. Beat in the yeast and quickly turn the dough out onto a marble slab or pastry board. Knead with greased hands until smooth. Put the dough into a bowl, cover with a cloth, and let rise in a warm place until doubled in bulk.

Heat 3 inches of oil, and fry walnut-sized pieces of the dough until golden brown. Take from the pan and drain on paper towels. Sprinkle with powdered sugar.

MAKES ABOUT 15 ZEPPOLI.

MAMMA'S CUSTARD—ITALIAN STYLE

My mom uses this basic recipe for cakes, puddings, and as the one Italian recipe that works great for English trifle. So get inventive! I'll bet you can come up with some terrific uses for it too.

1   *cup sugar*
2   *eggs*
½   *cup cornstarch*
1   *quart milk*
1   *tablespoon melted butter*
1   *teaspoon vanilla (or rum flavoring)*

In a saucepan blend sugar, eggs, and cornstarch, slowly adding the milk while stirring constantly over medium heat. Stir until just below boiling. Remove from heat, add 1 tablespoon of melted butter and the vanilla (or rum flavoring). Blend well.

Pour into dessert dishes and chill.

This custard is excellent as the center layer in a sponge cake. Spread it on cake while still warm. (See Mamma's Birthday Cake, page 211).

Variations: Add chocolate chips (about 6 ounces)—extra good—or add 6 ounces of melted unsweetened chocolate.

SERVES 6.

ZABAGLIONE (ITALIAN PUDDING)

If dessert could become a roving ambassador from Italy, zabaglione would be the number one candidate! It's considered *the* traditional Italian dessert and is famous throughout the world for its incredibly rich, frothy texture and amazing taste. It's fun to make, too!

6   *egg yolks*
6   *teaspoons sugar*
6   *tablespoons Amaretto or Marsala*
1   *tablespoon grated orange peel*
½   *cup whipping cream*

Combine egg yolks with sugar in top of double boiler and beat with a wire whisk until frothy. Add Amaretto or Marsala and grated orange peel. Place over gently boiling water and beat continuously until smooth. Remove from heat and place, still in boiler top, over ice cubes in bowl to cool. Then whip cream and fold into cool custard with a rubber spatula. Pour into individual serving cups and chill. Serve over poached pears or peaches, or as a layer in strawberry shortcake.

Variation: Sprinkle with shaved chocolate.

SERVES 4.

PEACHES IN RED WINE

Every kid feels there are certain things their parents do which embarrass them. Especially kids who are trying to be American, not Italian—like I was when I was growing up. When my father would eat big, ripe peaches with his homemade wine for dessert, it would make me so embarrassed! I thought this was definitely *not* a class act —even though I secretly loved the taste too. So you can imagine my surprise when, some years ago at a verrrrry fancy Italian restaurant, they served . . . you guessed it! Ripe peaches in red wine for dessert. Writing this book has helped me examine some of my attitudes toward my past. I wish that my father were alive today, because nothing would please me more than to take him to a fancy restaurant for Peaches in Red Wine.

really ripe freestone peaches, sliced
light red wine
candlelight

Put the peaches in wineglasses, pour the wine over them and let them sit for a while . . . just long enough for a father and son to talk awhile and get to know each other better. Try it out on your dad, I'm sure he'll like it.

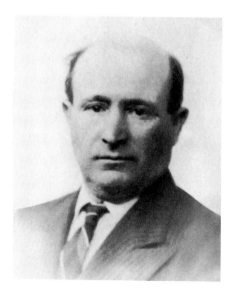

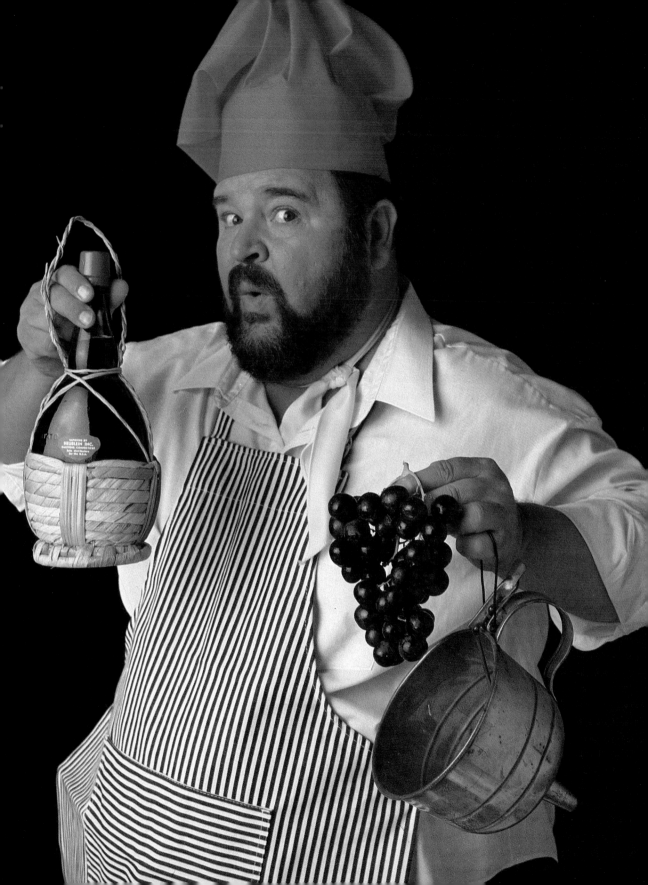

DIANE'S ANISE COOKIES

Every time I visit my mother in Brooklyn and we have an afternoon chat over coffee, my mom's neighbor, Diane, gently knocks on the door and comes in, always bringing some of these wonderful cookies on a plate. I call them "Diane's Cookies," and they are *fabulous*. (This is the one that sucks up the entire cup of coffee when you dunk it!)

2½ *cups sifted cake flour*
2   *teaspoons baking powder*
¼   *cup margarine*
1   *cup sugar*
4   *eggs*
1   *tablespoon anise extract*

Sift flour with the baking powder. In a medium bowl at medium speed, blend in the margarine with the sugar until very light. Add the eggs, one at a time, and beat after each addition. Add the flour mixture and beat at a low speed until blended.

Divide the mixture in half. Spread each half on a greased and floured cookie sheet, shaping each into an oval. Mold each oval into a mound: the sides low, the middle thick, and each oval about 12 inches long.

Bake for 20 minutes at 350 degrees, or until pale golden brown. Remove from the oven and cut into 1-inch slices . . . cut, cut, cut . . . cut. Turn each slice over on its side and you bake it another 10 to 15 minutes until it's golden brown.

What you have are crescent-shaped cookies. Let dry. After you've had a few bites of one, try dipping it in your coffee. It will shamelessly suck up the whole cup. Now you have to eat it fast, or the front end will fall into your coffee—then you're on your own.

MAKES ABOUT 20 COOKIES.

TESSIE'S RICE PUDDING

When I was working two shows a night at the Westbury Music Fair there was a wonderful, wild, and crazy lady named Tessie who fed me —and the entire cast and crew (among the hungriest people I'd ever met!)—some of the best meals ever. This particular recipe was everyone's favorite.

½ gallon milk
¼ pound butter
¾ cup sugar

Bring above to a slow boil.

Add:
1 cup rice

Lower flame to simmer and cook 45 minutes—stir often.

1 egg
½ pint heavy cream
1 teaspoon vanilla
1½ ounces Amaretto (optional)
cinnamon

Beat together the egg, cream, vanilla and Amaretto (if using) and add to the cooked rice. Mix thoroughly. Put in a serving dish and let cool. Sprinkle with cinnamon. Refrigerate.

SERVES 6–8.

PAULINE'S CINNAMON STICKS

Pauline Ossip works for my friend Father Orsini, and I guess God told her how to make these cookies, because they're sooooo good!

3   cups sugar
2   cups ground walnuts
1   tablespoon cinnamon
½   pound butter
½   pound cream cheese
2½   cups flour
1   egg, beaten

Mix together sugar, walnuts, and cinnamon and set aside. In another bowl, cream butter and cream cheese together. Add flour gradually. If dough is too soft, add a little more flour. Chill dough if you want to.

Roll dough out to ½ inch thick and spread the beaten egg all over the dough. Then use cinnamon mixture to cover dough. Cut into 1½-inch strips and twist.

Bake on a cookie sheet at 400 degrees for 8–10 minutes.

MAKES 50–60 CINNAMON STICKS.

EUGENE'S ALMOST NO FLOUR NUT CAKE

My sister has a friend named Eugene Canava, who brought this light, nutty, scrumptious cake to me and my mom, who flipped over it—*wow!* When my mom flips over somebody else's cooking, this is a special happening. Cut the finished cake into thin slices, and all you need is the time to enjoy its very individual taste. Serve it and just listen to the ooohs and ahhs!

1   dozen eggs, separated
¼   cup flour
½   teaspoon vanilla
½   teaspoon cinnamon
½   teaspoon lemon rind

2   teaspoons lemon juice
1   cup sugar
1   pound filberts (or walnuts or pecans), shelled and ground fine in food processor or grinder

Beat egg yolks with all the above ingredients except nuts, until smooth. Add nuts.

In a separate bowl, beat egg whites till stiff. Gently fold egg whites into above mixture.

Pour into greased Bundt pan and bake at 325 degrees for 1 hour and 10 minutes.

SERVES 8–10.

What Price Chocolate?

I remember when I was a kid we once got a year's supply of chocolate syrup and owed it all to a man with one leg. It was four o'clock one afternoon and a door-to-door salesman came to our house and asked Mamma if she wanted to buy chocolate syrup for the kids to mix with their milk after school. "Absolutely not!" she said. It was too expensive and they could drink the milk plain. Mamma asked him to please leave because there was no way she was going to buy the chocolate syrup. Then the man explained that he was trying to earn money for his family by selling chocolate syrup because he had lost a leg in the war. He said he found it hard to get a job. He stood up, put his left leg on a chair and pulled up his pants to reveal his wooden leg. He took out a penknife, stuck it in the calf of his wooden leg, and Mamma's eyes filled with tears. I knew that chocolate syrup was mine.

She bought six huge cans. Mamma said, "I mean, what else could I do? The poor man." I knew that guy had conned us, because when he put the penknife in his wooden leg, I could see lots of holes from past demonstrations. That leg had sold a lot of chocolate syrup. But Mamma was satisfied, that one-legged salesman was satisfied, and me . . . I was satisfied, too! Hee-hee.

If you love chocolate, then let me tell you—the following chocolate cake is to *die* for.

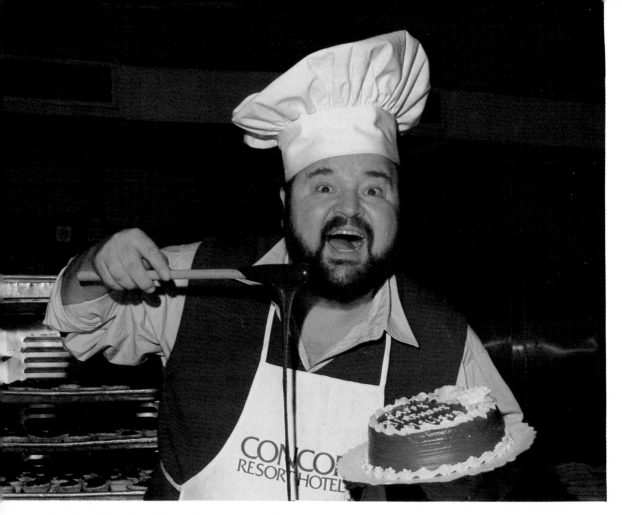

DEATH BY CHOCOLATE #1

    2 cups flour
    1 tablespoon double-acting baking powder
    ½ teaspoon baking soda
    2 cups sugar
    2 large eggs
    1 stick unsalted butter at room temperature, quartered
    1 cup sour cream
    ½ cup water
    2 teaspoons vanilla extract
    ½ cup plus 2 tablespoons cocoa
    1 12-oz. package semisweet chocolate chips
       powdered sugar
    1 Bundt pan

Sift flour, baking powder, and baking soda *twice*. Place in a small bowl. Beat the sugar and eggs in a large mixing bowl until sugar is dissolved. Add butter and mix into egg mixture thoroughly. Add sour cream, water, vanilla extract, and beat. Add flour mixture and cocoa and beat slowly just until flour is absorbed. Do not overbeat.

Fold in chocolate chips and pour into buttered Bundt pan. Bake at 350 degrees for 1 hour.

When cool, sift powdered sugar on top.

Variation: Replace ¼ cup of the water with Grand Marnier.

SERVES 8–10.

DEATH BY CHOCOLATE #2

I know I've taken a very strong position about fresh ingredients in my book, but this works beautifully for me when I'm pressed for time. And it's so good! If you won't tell, I won't tell.

4   *eggs*
1   *cup sour cream*
½   *cup water*
½   *cup oil*

Beat the above ingredients together in a large bowl until thoroughly mixed.

Add:

1   *chocolate cake mix*
1   *small box of instant chocolate pudding mix*

Beat until smooth.

Stir in:

1   *12-oz. package of semisweet chocolate chips*

Pour into buttered Bundt pan and bake at 350 degrees for 1 hour. When cool, sift powdered sugar on top.

Variation: Replace ¼ cup water with Grand Marnier.

SERVES 8–10.

CHOCOLATE TRUFFLE CAKE

And now from my old chocoholic beach buddy, Edna McHugh, another great recipe.

16   *ounces semisweet chocolate*
1   *stick unsalted butter*
1½   *teaspoons flour*
1½   *teaspoons sugar*
1   *teaspoon hot water*
4   *eggs, separated*
1   *cup whipping cream*

Preheat oven to 425 degrees. Grease bottom of 8-inch springform pan.

Melt chocolate and butter in the top of a double boiler. Remove from heat. Add flour, sugar, and water and blend well. Add egg yolks one at a time, beating well after each addition. In a separate bowl, beat egg whites until stiff, but not dry, and fold into the chocolate mixture.

Turn into pan and bake for *15 minutes only*.

Let cool completely, then chill in the refrigerator. Whip cream and spread over cake. Cut cake while cold, but let stand at room temperature for about 15 minutes before serving.

SERVES 8–10.

ANNE'S POUND CAKE

I am proud to have Jean Nidetch, founder of Weight Watchers, as a friend—she has inspired millions! At Weight Watchers we members have an opportunity to get up and discuss at length our problems with overeating. One time this little lady from New York stood up, and all she said was, "Sara Lee should drop dead!" I told that story on the Johnny Carson show and "Sara Lee" sent me two dozen pound cakes! Seriously, though, pound cake is another one of my favorites. I especially love the way my sister Anne makes it. She's got a recipe that's easy and great. Good enough for Sara Lee herself.

½   *cup of butter (room temperature)*
1   *cup of sugar*
2   *eggs*
½   *cup milk*
1   *teaspoon of vanilla*
1¾ *cups flour*
1   *heaping teaspoon baking powder*

Cream butter and sugar together. Then add eggs, milk, and vanilla. Beat lightly and gradually add flour and baking powder. Pour into a greased 9-inch loaf pan. Bake at 350 degrees for 45–50 minutes.

Variations on a Pound Cake
Variation #1:
2 *teaspoons sugar*
2 *teaspoons cinnamon*
4 *tablespoons chopped nuts*

Mix the three ingredients above together and sprinkle on top of cake before baking.

Variation #2: Add 1 cup of chopped walnuts or almonds to batter recipe.

Variation #3: Fold in 1 cup of blueberries before baking.

Variation #4: Add ½ cup of shredded coconut.

Variation #5: Fold in a cored, *chopped* apple before baking.

Variation #6: Fold in ½ cup of raisins before baking.

Variation #7: Put pineapple slices on the bottom of the pan. Pour the cake mixture over them and take 10 minutes off the baking time.

Variation #8: Place halved and pitted purple Italian plums cut side down in the pan. Sprinkle with 4 tablespoons of sugar and 1 tablespoon of cinnamon. Pour cake mixture over it, and also take 10 minutes off the baking time.

The variations stop here, but don't let your imagination quit!

MAKES 1 LOAF TO SERVE 8.

CREAMY CHEESECAKE

My assistant, Bette Adams, has been incredibly helpful to me with this cookbook. She loves to cook and have fun in the kitchen. Once when I was having a little get-together, Bette brought us this deliciously creamy cheesecake, and it's been a favorite of my kids ever since.

Crust:
¼   pound butter
1½ cups graham cracker crumbs
⅓   cup powdered sugar
½   cup crushed pecans

Melt butter and add to graham cracker crumbs, sugar and crushed pecans. Line bottom and sides of springform pan with the mixture, packing it down firmly.

Cheesecake Filling:
3 8-oz. packages cream cheese
1 cup granulated sugar
1 generous teaspoon vanilla
4 eggs

Put above ingredients into a food processor and mix well, using metal blade. Pour into springform pan and bake at 350 degrees for 50 minutes. Remove cheesecake. *Do not turn oven off.*

Topping:
Top with 1 pint of sour cream and return to oven for 5 more minutes.
  Let cool. Chill overnight.
  Serve with fresh strawberries or blueberries.

SERVES 8–10.

Too Much Water in the Orange Juice

Lately books have been written by the children of Joan Crawford, Bette Davis, Bing Crosby, even President Reagan, revealing harsh characteristics of these famous people in their role as parents. I was sitting at the breakfast table with Peter, Michael, and David, and I protested that it was unfair to write about famous parents and depict them in an unfavorable light. I asked my three sons straight out if they thought I was ever unfair. They unanimously said yes, that I was indeed unfair, scary at times, that I yelled and scolded, and that I was not the incredibly warm, sweet, loving, wonderful, gentle, and always kind father I thought I was. Michael took the opportunity to remind me that I used four cans of water instead of three when I made the frozen orange juice. Everyone at the breakfast table laughed and cheered in agreement . . . which I thought was cruel. I warned my children that if they wrote about me, I would come back and haunt them.

The next day, Michael and David were having a huge argument in the front hall. I stepped between them and sent them in opposite directions—David to the patio, and Michael to his room. Michael took three steps, stopped, turned, and pointed his finger at me and said, "It's going in the book!" I know that I'm going to go down in history as the inconsiderate father who put too much water in the orange juice. I know it! Look, you just can't win. Here's a recipe for my sister Anne's Orange Juice Cookies, and they *are* winners!

SISTER ANNE'S ORANGE JUICE COOKIES

I have a favorite sister, Anne. She is also my only sister. I also have three sons who have a favorite cookie, especially with their favorite glass of milk.

⅓	cup sugar	3	cups flour
1½	sticks margarine	3	teaspoons baking powder
3	eggs		
1	teaspoon vanilla		
½	cup orange juice		

Blend the first 5 ingredients in a blender and pour into a bowl. Add the flour and baking powder and knead *very thoroughly*. Batter must not be sticky . . . may require more flour.

After nicely blended, take a large tablespoon of batter (or a walnut-size amount) and roll between your hands to form a long pretzel-like stick. You may make cookies in this shape, or bring 2 ends together to form a small doughnut, or press into flat cookie shapes.

Preheat oven to 350 degrees. Place cookies on a large, ungreased cookie sheet. Let stand 10 minutes at room temperature before baking. Bake for 15–17 minutes until lightly golden brown.

Icing (prepare while cookies are baking):
½ *pound confectioners' sugar*
½ *cup orange juice*
½ *teaspoon vanilla*

Put all ingredients in a mixing bowl and blend until you get the consistency of a heavy syrup. If necessary, add more orange juice sparingly. When cookies are done, dip each hot cookie into the icing mixture, which will form a glaze over the cookies. Place on a dish. Sprinkle with candy confetti. Let cool until icing dries . . . *and enjoy!*

MAKES 24 COOKIES.

(Have some with your kids, while you tell them you love them.) Peter, Michael, David . . . I love you with all my heart!

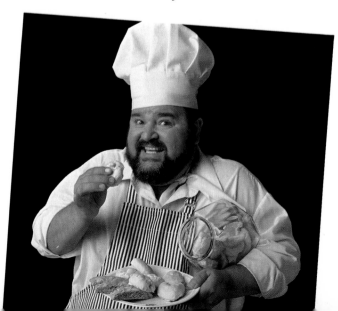

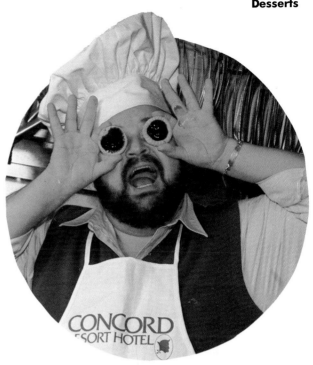

DOM'S NO SUGAR BAKED APPLES

From the days at Weight Watchers—and still great—a standard in
my home.

6   *Pippin or any tart, firm apples (leave skin on), cored and sliced*
½   *cup raisins*
½   *cup walnuts, chopped*
1   *teaspoon cinnamon*
½   *cup Grape-Nuts*
1   *cup apple juice*

Cover the bottom of a baking dish with the apples. Distribute raisins
and walnuts evenly over the apples. Sprinkle lightly with cinnamon.
Top with Grape-Nuts. Dribble the apple juice over the Grape-Nuts,
and bake in a 350-degree oven for 1 hour.
    Wonderful with whipped cream, yogurt or ice cream.

SERVES 4–6.

Writing this book has been a real gas for me. I've thoroughly enjoyed collecting all these recipes. But more fun than that was collecting all the memories—it was lovely for me to have all those extra conversations with my mom . . . who I thank from the bottom of my heart. For me the whole experience was like a toast to life. Remembering the past and sharing our "pasta" inventions really brought us so much closer. I will always be grateful to Simon and Schuster for that. My mom has a very nurturing nature, and I can see that I'm the same way—I like to make people comfortable, especially when they visit my home. When they come to dinner, walk in the door and say they love the smell . . . "What's cooking?" *I like that!* I like when large crowds come over for the holidays—I get to use my big platters! And no matter how much food I've cooked I invariably think, "I hope there's enough." So if someday you find yourself at our dinner table, don't be surprised if I turn to you and say, just like my mamma did, "Eat this . . . it'll make you feel better."

Salute! To life!

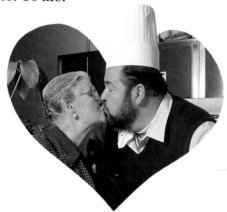

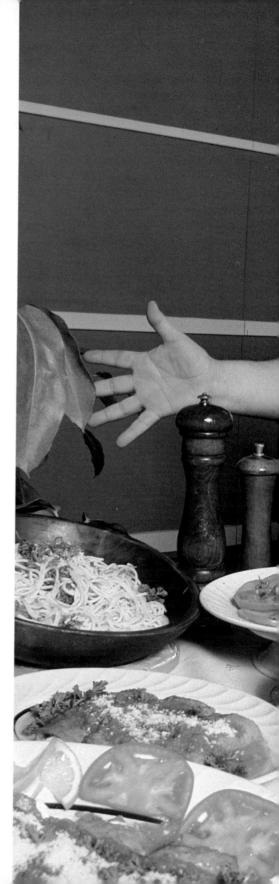

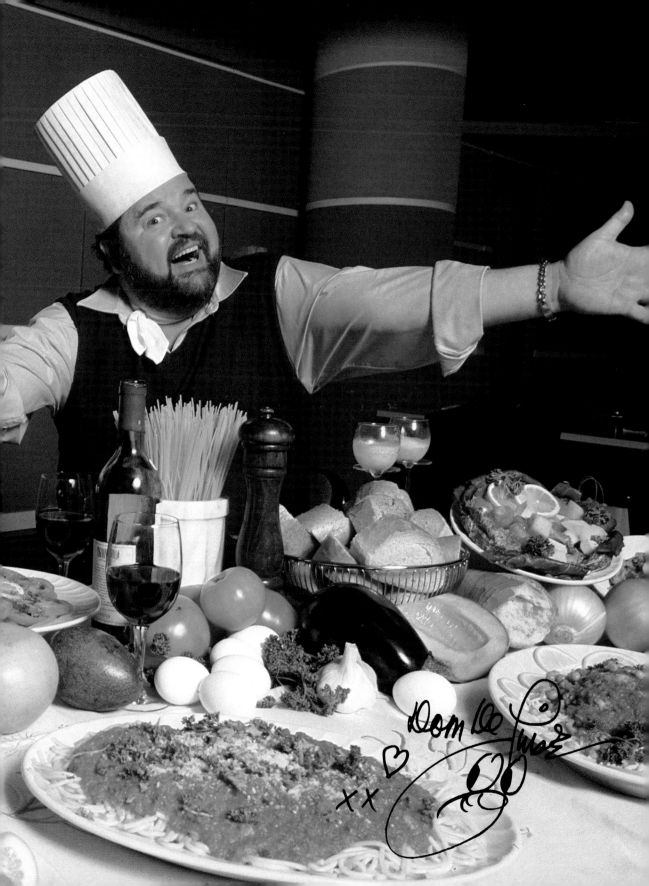

INDEX

aglio e olio, Dom's, 124
angel hair with white clam sauce
    à la Peggy, 130
anise cookies, Diane's, 220
Anna Banana's Italian sausage
    pie, 67
Anna Maria Italiano's potatoes
    and fagioli, 76–77
Anne Bancroft's vegetarian chili,
    78
Anne's orange juice cookies,
    Sister, 229–30
Anne's pound cake, 226–27
Anne's string beans, my sister,
    75
Anne's stuffed mushrooms, my
    sister, 93
apples, baked, Dom's no sugar,
    231–32
artichoke hearts, 51
    frittata, 66
artichokes, stuffed, 80
asparagus salad, East-West,
    58
Aunt Rose's zucchini bread,
    206

baked apples, Dom's no sugar,
    231–32
baked clams, 184
barley mushroom soup, Julann's
    fat-free hearty, 41
basic polenta, 143
Battista, pesto alla, 110
beans, cannellini:
    and escarole soup, 30
    Mamma's pasta e fagioli, 85
    and potatoes, Anna Maria
        Italiano's, 76–77
beans, kidney, in Anne
        Bancroft's vegetarian chili,
        78

beans, string, my sister Anne's,
    75
bean threads, deep-fried, 53
beef:
    Dinah's moussaka, 175–77
    Dom's Mom's meatballs, 164–65
    Mamma's (and Michael's) meat
        sauce, 122
    Mamma's Sunday sauce, 118
    stew, Burt's, 167–68
beer bread, Mary Daurio's,
    206–7
bouillabaisse, 190–91
braided egg bread, Mamma's,
    199
bread, 194–207
    Aunt Rose's zucchini, 206
    cheese and onion, 202
    loaves and fishes, 193
    Mamma's braided egg, 199
    Mamma's Easter papoose,
        197–98
    Mary Daurio's beer, 206–7
    Mom's sausage, 200
    pizza dough, 207
    pumpkin, in a coffee can
        telephone, 201–2
breakfast foods:
    grains, 142–43
    Italian scramble, 63
broccoli with rigatoni, 107
broth, Mamma's spinach and
        potatoes in, 74
brown rice Louise, 142

cabbage, Chinese, in Dom's
        steamed dumplings, 166
Caesar salad, Dom's, 52
cakes:
    chocolate truffle, 226
    Eugene's almost no flour nut,
        222–23

Mamma's happy birthday,
        anniversary, and wedding,
        211–12
    pound, Anne's, 226–27
calamari (squid):
    Mamma's Italian fish stew, 180
    salad of the sea, 182–83
    and shellfish sauce, 133–34
    stuffed, 183
cannellini beans, see beans,
    cannellini
Carol Burnett's scampi, 186–187
cheese:
    Anna Banana's Italian sausage
        pie, 67
    artichoke frittata, 66
    chicken (easy does it) sauce,
        126
    Dom's eggs alla diavolo,
        64
    Dom's Mom's stuffed eggplant
        rolls, 87
    eggplant-stuffed peppers, 88
    frittata for Julia Child, 65
    gnocchi #1, 105
    gnocchi verdi, 106–7
    Italian scramble, 63
    lasagne, 113
    mozzarella and tomato salad,
        49
    and onion bread, 202
cheesecake, creamy, 228
chicken:
    Dominick, 149
    Dom's ginger, 152
    Georgiana's tortilla soup, 40
    Mamma's, 148
    Maria's paella, 153
    Nancy Reagan's Baja
        California, 150
    and/or rabbit, Italian fried, 154
    salad, Dom's Chinese, 53–55

(easy does it) sauce, 126
with wild rice, Loni's, 150–151
chili, Anne Bancroft's
  vegetarian, 78
Chinese chicken salad, Dom's,
  53–55
chocolate:
  death by, #1, 224–25
  death by, #2, 225
  truffle cake, 226
chowder, Mel Brooks' red clam,
  36–37
cinnamon sticks, Pauline's, 222
clam(s):
  baked, 184
  bouillabaisse, 190–91
  calamari and shellfish sauce,
    133–34
  chowder, Mel Brooks' red, 36–
    37
  Mamma's seafood sauce, 132
  Maria's paella, 153
  sauce, red, for Dino, 128–129
  sauce, white, à la Peggy, 130
cod, in Mamma's Italian fish
  stew, 180
cookies:
  Diane's anise, 220
  Sister Anne's orange juice,
    229–30
creamy cheesecake, 228
crispelle, 213
croquettes, Vincenza's egg, 69
crust, pie, 67
custard Italian style, Mamma's,
  216
cutlets, Mamma's veal, 173

death by chocolate #1, 224–225
death by chocolate #2, 225
deep-fried bean threads or rice
  sticks, 53
desserts, 208–32
  anise cookies, Diane's, 220
  apples, Dom's no sugar baked,
    231–32
  cake, Mamma's happy
    birthday, anniversary, and
    wedding, 211–12
  cheesecake, creamy, 228
  chocolate truffle cake, 226
  cinnamon sticks, Pauline's, 222
  crispelle, 213
  custard—Italian style,
    Mamma's, 216
  death by chocolate #1, 224–25
  death by chocolate #2,
    225
  grain pie, Mom's Easter, 215

nut cake, Eugene's almost no
  flour, 222–23
orange juice cookies, Sister
  Anne's, 229–30
pound cake, Anne's, 226–227
pudding, Italian, 217
rice pudding, Tessie's, 221
strufoli, 214
zabaglione, 217
zeppoli, 216
Diane's anise cookies, 220
Dinah's moussaka, 175–77
Dino, red clam sauce for, 128
dough, pizza, 207
dressing:
  Dom's Chinese chicken salad,
    54–55
  my Italian style vinaigrette, 59
  for summer salad, 57
dumplings, Dom's steamed, 166

Easter grain pie, Mom's, 215
Easter papoose bread, Mamma's,
  197–98
East-West asparagus salad, 58
egg(s):
  alla diavolo, Dom's, 64
  artichoke frittata, 66
  braided bread, Mamma's, 199
  croquettes, Vincenza's, 69
  frittata for Julia Child, 65
  Italian scramble, 63
  pasta for ravioli or manicotti,
    104
eggplant(s):
  balls, Father Orsini's, 90–91
  Dinah's moussaka, 175–77
  everybody's pot le gel, 95
  rolls, stuffed, Dom's Mom's, 87
  sandwich, open-faced, 90
  sauce, Mamma's, 127
  stuffed peppers, 88
escarole:
  and beans soup, 30
  soup, Mamma's, 29
Eugene's almost no flour nut
  cake, 222–23

fagioli:
  e pasta, Mamma's, 85
  and potatoes, Anna Maria
    Italiano's, 76
fat-free hearty mushroom barley
  soup, Julann's, 41
Father Orsini's eggplant balls,
  90–92
fish, 178–93
  bouillabaisse, 190–91
  calamari, stuffed, 183

and loaves, 193
pasta salad, Dom's, 56
redfish, Chef Paul
  Prudhomme's blackened,
  191–93
salad of the sea, 182–83
sauce, Mamma's, 132
sole, Dom's stuffed, 189
soup, Mamma's Friday night
  hearty, 34–35
stew, Mamma's Italian,
  188
see also shellfish
fresh pasta, 103
fried rabbit and/or chicken,
  Italian, 154
frittata, artichoke, 66
frittata for Julia Child, 65

garlic and oil, 124
gazpacho, 38
Georgiana's tortilla soup, 40
ginger chicken, Dom's, 152
gnocchi:
  #1, 105
  #2, 105–6
  verdi, 106–7
grain(s):
  basic polenta, 143
  breakfast, lunch, dinner, 142–
    143
  pie, Mom's Easter, 215

halibut:
  bouillabaisse, 190–91
  Mamma's Friday night hearty
    fish soup, 34–35
happy birthday, anniversary, and
  wedding cake, Mamma's,
  211–12
harlot sauce, 125

Italian (style):
  fish stew, Mamma's, 188
  fried rabbit and/or chicken,
    154
  Mamma's custard, 216
  my vinaigrette dressing, 59
  pudding, 217
  scramble, 63
Italian sausage:
  bread, Mom's, 200
  Mamma's homemade, 163–164
  Mamma's spaghetti sauce with,
    123
  Mamma's Sunday sauce, 118
  Maria's paella, 153
  pie, Anna Banana's, 67
  with peppers and onions, 162

Julann's fat-free hearty
    mushroom barley soup, 41
Julia Child, frittata for, 65

kidney beans, in Anne Bancroft's
    vegetarian chili, 78

lamb, in Dinah's moussaka, 175–
    177
lasagne, 113
lentil soup, Mamma's, 30–31
linguine, sauces for:
    calamari and shellfish, 133–134
    scandalous scallop, 134–35
    white clam, à la Peggy,
        130
loaves and fishes, 193
lobster bouillabaisse, 190–91

manicotti, egg pasta for, 104
marinara sauce, Mamma's, 120–
    121
Marsala veal, Mamma's, 169–
    170
Mary Daurio's beer bread, 206–7
Ma Ziti's stuffed shells, 114–115
meat, 159–77
    beef stew, Burt's, 167–68
    dumplings, Dom's steamed,
        166
    moussaka, Dinah's, 175–77
    paella, Maria's, 153
    sauce, Mamma's (and
        Michael's), 122
    sauce, Mamma's Sunday, 118
    sausage, Mamma's homemade,
        163–64
    sausage bread, Mom's, 200
    sausage pie, Anna Banana's
        Italian, 67
    sausages with peppers and
        onions, 162
    veal, stuffed breast of, 174
    veal cutlets, Mamma's, 173
    veal Marsala, Mamma's, 169–
        170
    veal piccata, 173
meatballs:
    Dom's Mom's, 164–65
    Mamma's stracciatelle with
        tiny, 32
Mel Brook's red clam chowder,
    36–37
Montalban salad, 50
Monterey Jack, in frittata for
    Julia Child, 65
mostaccioli, Mom's mussels
    marinara with, 131
moussaka, Dinah's, 175–77

mozzarella:
    artichoke frittata, 66
    Dom's Mom's stuffed eggplant
        rolls, 87
    eggplant-stuffed peppers, 88
    frittata for Julia Child, 65
mushroom(s):
    barley soup, Julann's fat-free
        hearty, 41
    Dom's stuffed, 92–93
    Mamma's stuffed, 92
    my sister Anne's stuffed, 93
mussels:
    Mamma's, 185
    Maria's paella, 153
    marinara with mostaccioli,
        Mom's, 131

Nancy Reagan's onion wine soup,
    45
nut cake, Eugene's almost no
    flour, 222–23

oil and garlic, 124
onion(s):
    and cheese bread, 202
    and peppers, sausages with,
        162
    wine soup, Nancy Reagan's, 45
open-faced eggplant sandwich, 90
orange juice cookies, Sister
    Anne's, 229–30

paella, Maria's, 153
Parmesan, in chicken (easy does
    it) sauce, 126
pasta, 99–115
    aglio e olio, Dom's, 124
    broccoli with rigatoni, 107
    calamari and shellfish sauce,
        133–34
    chicken (easy does it) sauce,
        126
    Dom's seafood salad, 56
    egg, for ravioli or manicotti,
        104
    e fagioli, Mamma's, 85
    fresh, 103
    gnocchi #1, 105
    gnocchi #2, 105–6
    gnocchi verdi, 106–7
    lasagne, 113
    Lucy's, 108
    Mamma's seafood sauce, 132
    Ma Ziti's stuffed shells, 114–
        115
    Mom's mussels marinara with
        mostaccioli, 131
    pesto alla Battista, 110

    scandalous scallop sauce, 134–
        135
    spinach, 104
    white clam sauce à la Peggy,
        130
Pauline's cinnamon sticks, 222
Paul Prudhomme's blackened
    redfish, 191–93
peaches in red wine, 218
peppers, bell:
    eggplant-stuffed, 88
    like you've never had them
        before!, 79
    and onions, sausages with, 162
pesto alla Battista, 110
piccata, veal, 173–74
pie, Mom's Easter grain, 215
piecrust, 67
pizza:
    dough, 207
    grana, 215
polenta:
    basic, 143
    rabbit con, 157
pork:
    Dom's Mom's meatballs, 164–
        165
    Dom's steamed dumplings,
        166
    Mamma's homemade sausage,
        163–64
    Mamma's Sunday sauce, 118
potato(es):
    and fagioli, Anna Maria
        Italiano's, 76
    gnocchi #2, 105–6
    rice soup, 33
    and spinach in broth,
        Mamma's, 74
pot le gel, everybody's, 95
poultry, see chicken
pound cake, Anne's, 226–27
prawns, in Carol Burnett's
    scampi, 186–87
primavera:
    Dom's, 109
    risotto, 141
pudding:
    Italian, 217
    Tessie's rice, 221
pumpkin bread in a coffee can
    telephone, 201–2
puttanesca sauce, 125

rabbit, 154–57
    cacciatore, 155
    and/or chicken, Italian fried,
        154
    con polenta, 157

ratatouille, 89
ravioli, egg pasta for, 104
red clam chowder, Mel Brooks', 36–37
red clam sauce for Dino, 128–129
redfish, Chef Paul Prudhomme's blackened, 191–93
red peppers like you've never had them before!, 79
red snapper, in Mamma's Italian fish stew, 180
red wine, peaches in, 218
rice, 136–43
    brown, Louise, 142
    potato soup, 33
    risotto, 140
    risotto primavera, 141
    sticks, deep-fried, 53
    wild, Loni's chicken with, 150–151
rice pudding, Tessie's, 221
rigatoni, broccoli with, 107
risotto, 140
    primavera, 141
Rita's recipe from Felina in Italy, 90
rolls, Dom's Mom's stuffed eggplant, 87
Rose's zucchini bread, 206

salads, 46–59
    Caesar, Dom's, 52
    Dom's Chinese chicken, 53–55
    Dom's seafood pasta, 56
    East-West asparagus, 58
    Salvatore's sister Sally's sensational summer, 56
    of the sea, 182–83
    tomato and mozzarella, 49
    viva Montalban, 50
Salvatore's sister Sally's sensational summer salad, 56–57
sandwich, open-faced eggplant, 90
sauces, 117–35
    chicken (easy does it), 126
    garlic and oil, 124
    white clam, à la Peggy, 130
sauces, tomato:
    calamari and shellfish, 133–134
    chicken (easy does it), 126
    eggplant, Mamma's, 127
    Mamma's (and Michael's), 122
    Mamma's Sunday, 118
    marinara, Mamma's, 120–121
    puttanesca, 125
    red clam, for Dino, 128–29
    scandalous scallop, 134–35

seafood, Mamma's, 132
spaghetti, with Italian sausage, Mamma's, 123
sausage, Italian:
    bread, Mom's, 200
    Mamma's homemade, 163–164
    Mamma's spaghetti sauce with, 123
    Mamma's Sunday sauce, 118
    Maria's paella, 153
    pie, Anna Banana's, 67
    with peppers and onions, 162
scallop(s):
    bouillabaisse, 190–91
    Mamma's Italian fish stew, 180
    Mamma's seafood sauce, 132
    sauce, scandalous, 134–35
scramble, Italian, 63
seasoning mix for Chef Paul Prudhomme's blackened redfish, 191–93
shellfish:
    bouillabaisse, 190–91
    and calamari sauce, 133–134
    clam chowder, Mel Brook's red, 36–37
    clams, baked, 184
    clam sauce à la Peggy, white, 130
    loaves and fishes, 193
    Mamma's Italian fish stew, 188
    Mamma's seafood sauce, 132
    Maria's paella, 153
    mussels, Mamma's, 185
    mussels marinara with mostaccioli, Mom's, 131
    salad of the sea, 182–83
    scallop sauce, scandalous, 134–135
    scampi, Carol Burnett, 186–87
shells, Ma Ziti's stuffed, 114–115
shrimp:
    bouillabaisse, 190–91
    calamari and shellfish sauce, 133–34
    Carol Burnett's scampi, 186–87
    Mamma's Italian fish stew, 180
    Mamma's seafood sauce, 132
    Maria's paella, 153
    salad of the sea, 182–83
Sister Anne's orange juice cookies, 229–30
Sister Anne's string beans, 75
Sister Anne's stuffed mushrooms, 93
snapper, red, in Mamma's Friday night hearty fish soup, 34

sole:
    Dom's stuffed, 189
    Mamma's Friday night hearty fish soup, 34
soups, 27–45
    beef stew, Burt's, 167–68
    clam chowder, Mel Brooks' red, 36–37
    escarole, Mamma's, 29
    escarole and beans, 30
    fish, Mamma's Friday night hearty, 34–35
    gazpacho, 38
    lentil, Mamma's, 30–31
    mushroom barley, Julann's fat-free hearty, 41
    onion wine, Nancy Reagan's, 45
    potato rice, 33
    rabbit stew, stewed, 156
    stracciatelle with tiny meatballs, Mamma's, 32
    tortilla, Georgiana's, 40
    vegetable stew, 73
    Veronica's lake, 34
spaghetti sauces:
    chicken (easy does it), 126
    with Italian sausage, Mamma's, 123
spinach:
    gnocchi verdi, 106–7
    pasta, 104
    and potatoes in broth, Mamma's, 74
    rolls, Mamma's, 94
squid (calamari):
    Mamma's Italian fish stew, 180
    salad of the sea, 182–83
    and shellfish sauce, 133–34
    stuffed, 183
steamed dumplings, Dom's, 166
stews:
    Burt's beef, 167–68
    Mamma's Italian fish, 188
    stewed rabbit, 156
    vegetable, 73
stock, fish, for bouillabaisse, 190
stracciatelle with tiny meatballs, Mamma's, 32
string beans, my sister Anne's, 75
strufoli, 214
stuffed:
    artichokes, 80
    breast of veal, 174
    calamari, 183
    eggplant rolls, Dom's Mom's, 87
    mushrooms, Dom's, 92–93
    mushrooms, Mamma's, 92

stuffed (*cont.*)
  mushrooms, my sister Anne's, 93
  peppers, eggplant-, 88
  shells, Ma Ziti's, 114–15
Sunday sauce, Mamma's, 118

Tessie's rice puding, 221
tomato and mozzarella salad, 49
tomato sauces, *see* sauces, tomato
tortilla soup, Georgiana's, 40
turkey, in Dom's steamed dumplings, 166

veal:
  cutlets, Mamma's, 173
  Marsala, Mamma's, 169–70
  piccata, 173–74
  stuffed breast of, 174
vegetable(s):
  artichoke frittata, 66
  artichoke hearts, 51
  artichokes, stuffed, 80
  broccoli with rigatoni, 107
  eggplant balls, Father Orsini's, 90–92
  eggplant rolls, Dom's Mom's stuffed, 87

eggplant sandwich, open-faced, 90
eggplant sauce, Mamma's, 127
eggplant-stuffed peppers, 88
escarole and beans, 30
gazpacho, 38
gnocchi verdi, 106–7
Italian scramble, 63
moussaka, Dinah's, 175–77
mushroom barley soup, Julann's fat-free hearty, 41
mushrooms, Mamma's stuffed, 92
mushrooms, my sister Anne's stuffed, 93
paella, Maria's, 153
peppers and onions, sausages with, 162
potatoes and fagioli, Anna Maria Italiano's, 76
pot le gel, everybody's, 95
primavera, Dom's, 109
ratatouille, 89
red peppers like you've never had them before!, 79
risotto primavera, 141
soup, Georgiana's tortilla, 40
spinach and potatoes in broth, Mamma's, 74

spinach pasta, 104
spinach rolls, Mamma's, 94
stew, 73
string beans, my sister Anne's, 75
vegetarian chili, Anne Bancroft's, 78
Veronica's lake, 34
zucchini bread, Aunt Rose's, 206
see also salads; tomato sauces
vinaigrette dressing, my Italian style, 59
Vincenza's egg croquettes, 69
viva Montalban salad, 50

white clam sauce à la Peggy, 130
wild rice, Loni's chicken with, 150–51
wine, peaches in red, 218
wine onion soup, Nancy Reagan's, 45

zabaglione, 217
zeppoli, 216
ziti shells, Ma Ziti's stuffed, 114–115
zucchini bread, Aunt Rose's, 206

PHOTO CREDITS

KITCHENWARE CREDITS

About the Author

Dom DeLuise is one of America's best-loved comedians. He has appeared in four Mel Brooks movies, *The Twelve Chairs*, *Blazing Saddles*, *Silent Movie*, and *The History of the World—Part I*. Along with Gene Wilder, Dom has filmed *The Adventures of Sherlock Holmes' Smarter Brother*, *The World's Greatest Lover*, and *Haunted Honeymoon*.

He has made six films with Burt Reynolds, *Silent Movie*, *The End*, *Smokey and the Bandit II*, *Cannonball Run I* and *II*, and *The Best Little Whorehouse in Texas*.

DeLuise has worked with Dean Martin, Sammy Davis, Jr., Telly Savalas, Shirley MacLaine, Liza Minnelli, Henry Fonda, Jack Benny, Peter Sellers, Jimmy Stewart, Sid Caesar, Jim Nabors, Ricardo Montalban, and Frank Sinatra, to name only a few.

Mr. DeLuise became a household face when television viewers saw him daily for many years as the spokesman for NCR and Ziploc. He lives in California with his actress wife, Carol Arthur, a dog, a cat, a bird, and their three children, Peter, Michael, and David—who all have their talented eyes on show business. All the sons complain because their father is always saying, "Eat this . . . it'll make you feel better."

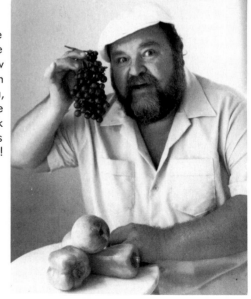

Regina DeLuise's works are represented in the collections of the Art Institute in Chicago, the Metropolitan and the Museum of Modern Art in New York, and the Canadian Centre for Architecture in Montreal. She has exhibited in New York, California, Chicago, and Italy, where she traveled with the author of this book. Fifteen minutes after she took this picture, the grapes disappeared. She thinks Uncle Dom did it!